MICHAEL SCOFIELD

PERFECT SELF CONTROL

WELLBEING FOR 110 YEARS

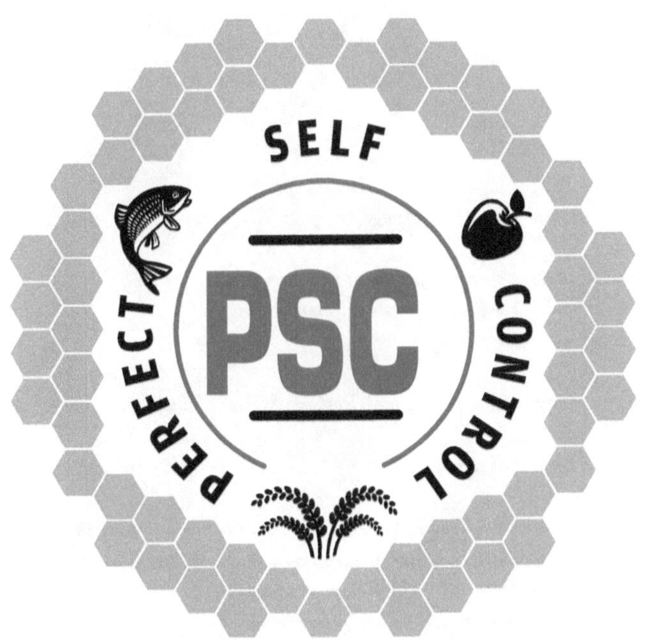

authorHOUSE®

AuthorHouse™ UK
1663 Liberty Drive
Bloomington, IN 47403 USA
www.authorhouse.co.uk
Phone: UK TFN: 0800 0148641 (Toll Free inside the UK)
*   UK Local: 02036 956322 (+44 20 3695 6322 from outside the UK)*

Published by AuthorHouse 08/17/2020

ISBN: 978-1-7283-5586-3 (sc)
ISBN: 978-1-7283-5585-6 (e)

CONTENTS

Dear Reader,

You have made the best decision of your life in buying this book! This book summarizes 30 years of learning, data collection, lengthy meditations and experiments which have been conducted on myself. It provides you with the key to a healthy, happy, energetic and successful life, which could last you 110-120 years depending on your genes.

Perfect Self Control is a nutritional system that optimizes your metabolism, recommending only those nutriments your body requires at specific times of the day. By applying PSC, you can lengthen the lifetime of your cells, thereby extending your body's lifetime as well.

The first step is to understand the core principles of healthy nutrition, and then you need to introduce these principles to your diet in order to enjoy the above-mentioned benefits. It is a complicated and complex task to find the really healthy diet for a specific person. This is why I have tried to create a brief and comprehensible guide, supporting you to attain a clear understanding of it.

There are plenty of misconceptions and half-truths in people's understanding of this topic. We are given conflicting advice. Some advise us to go vegan since meat is acidic and contributes to high cholesterol levels. Then another source will tell us we should always eat meat since our ancestors thrived on it, but we should also eat wholegrain seeds. Some people are tirelessly trying to convince us to take certain medicines and vitamins. I have even heard of a diet suggesting a tomato-only week!

In order to be healthy and maintain a good weight, you don't need to self-torture or endure a heavy diet. Moreover, you must enjoy your food! It is crucial to introduce a varied diet, based on certain foods that are healthy for you, and eating only until your stomach is full. Yes, as you can see, even if you are attempting to lose weight, you should still eat proper meals. However, you have to gently introduce a new system to your daily and weekly diet. While preparing your meals, pay attention to choosing fresh, tasty and high-quality ingredients since they form the basis of a delicious and healthy meal. Due to the biorhythm of the cells in our body, we need different nutrition at different times of the day. We need carbohydrates during the day and proteins in the evening. This is why it is important to have the right meals at different times of the day.

For an effective digestive system, we have to pay attention how we pair certain ingredients together. Besides nutrition, there are other factors affecting our health, but nutrition is the most important factor, determining our health at 80-90%.

"You become what you eat," said Hippocrates in ancient Greece. As the leader of the School of Kos, he taught his pupils that the source of disease is unhealthy nutrition. He is also famous for his quote, "Let food be the medicine and medicine be the food." That is why the timing of suitable meals is of utmost importance.

According to a Buddhist monk, "There is only a single way things can be." There is only one truth, not another. The truth can be complicated, but there is only one, so if you desire an answer for what is the perfect diet for you, there is only one true answer.

There are two ways to obtain this answer. We can examine the functioning of your metabolism, including digestion and different kinds of biochemical processes. Thus, by inspecting the weaknesses of your metabolism, it becomes possible to avoid its obstacles and improve its functioning.

There is another way: we can study how our ancestors lived and nourished their bodies at different times of the day, as their digestive system, body type, and biorhythm adapted to accessible foods and specific environmental challenges through human evolution. As we carry their genes, by tracing back their lifestyle and nutriments, we have the potential to find out the most suitable diet for you.

The last three hundred years, which have brought numerous significant changes to the dietary customs of the human race, is a relatively short period compared to the last two million years in the history of mankind. Consequently, the genes of the human race have not adapted well to the changed new diet so the physical state of mankind has deteriorated vastly. This is the result of the exponential advances originating from the technological revolution.

Through modern milling, removing bran and germ from grain, we are able to consume refined grains instead of whole grains. However, this is not all: it also removes from our diet essential sources of vitamin B and fiber, which are crucial for digestion. Processed foodstuffs abound with genetically modified organisms, (or GMO), artificial colorings, additives and preservatives. These materials are toxic, carcinogenic and acidifying. Aside from this, processed foods lack enzymes and vitamins necessary for normal bodily functions.

As a consequence of the invention of the refrigerator and food canning, the natural biorhythm of people is disrupted. Nowadays people commonly access any food at any time, even food that spoils very fast without refrigeration.

The reason we should avoid having processed foods is that the additives and preservatives in them are toxic for us. On packaged food labels, these are usually identified by a capital E, such as E-189. Always prepare your food using fresh and unprocessed ingredients! They are cheaper, tastier and healthier. There are foodstuffs that your ancestors have never encountered or consumed, therefore neither they nor you have the enzymes required to break them down; hence you cannot digest and utilize them. Moreover, they are not only indigestible, but also specifically harmful for you. Their long-term consumption can cause obesity, allergies, type 2 diabetes, cardiovascular diseases and cancer.

There are foods that are harmful per se, regardless if they are organic or unprocessed. You must stay away from eating them! It is important to know who we really are, what are our strengths and weaknesses.

From a genetic perspective, four different kinds of people have evolved from our early ancestors. This is not about race or skin color, as they are irrelevant differences in terms of human genetics.

The invention of high-resolution microscopes have enabled scientists to analyse human blood. It was discovered that the blood cells of different people can differ substantially. Four types were identified, namely blood type (or group) O, A, B, and AB. First, it was assumed that the differences were superficial, including only blood cells. Nowadays we are aware that people of different blood groups have different genes, digestive systems, musculature, nervous systems and temperament. This is why organ transplantation is possible only within the same blood type.

Each of them is differently affected by particular types of food. Blood groups are determined by the DNA encoded in dominant genes, such as A or B, overwriting type O recessive genes. This book will elaborate on the above and educate you to be able to live your best possible and most healthy and long lifestyle.

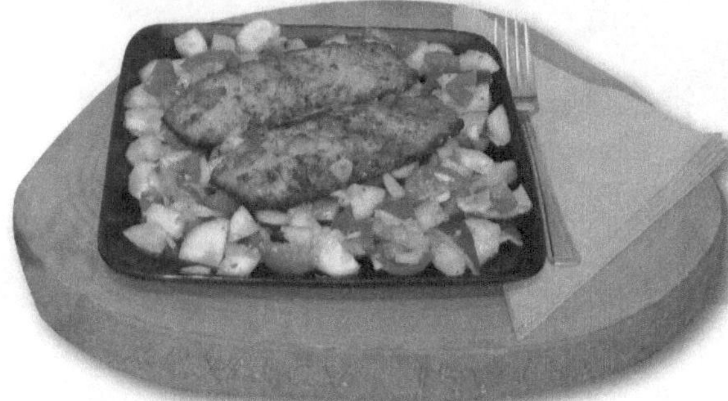

Human Life and Development Before the Civilization Revolution

Plenty of artifacts have been excavated and the science of genetics has evolved in recent years, providing evidence for millions of years of human development and behaviour. Therefore, we have sufficient knowledge about our ancestor's tools and their functions, as well as about how, when and what they hunted, fished and gathered, and how they used fire for protection and cooking.

We have obtained precise information on foods consumed by cavemen as well as by the wild environment surrounding them, enabling the reconstruction of their everyday lives. We know that our ancestors formed little groups as families grew, obtaining food by hunting, fishing and gathering. Originating in Africa, they gradually populated the whole Earth. They were surrounded by predators that hunted from dusk to dawn. To avoid becoming prey themselves, our ancestors had to empty their hunting traps and nets before dusk, as predators were starving for their catches and prey.

With fresh kill in their hands, the hunters and fishermen went back to their camps as quickly as possible. They needed the protection of fire to skin and gut the kill, as they were surrounded by predators becoming excited by the smell of blood. So fire was set in a pit, and they wrapped fish or meat and edible innards together with hard root vegetables (e.g. carrot, celery and beetroot) into large leaves. These packs of food were put onto the embers, covered by leaves, and left there for several hours to roast.

Their appetites were satisfied by this delicious dinner in the early evening hours. Hunters and other males had the privilege to eat first, the rest of the community ate after. When everybody was full - which was a rare occasion - the remaining food was consumed by dogs and cats. As refrigeration was unknown, leaving roast meat and fish was undoubtedly impractical as it would have been quickly spoiled in warm climates and predators would have been attracted by the smell while people were sleeping. So, after din-

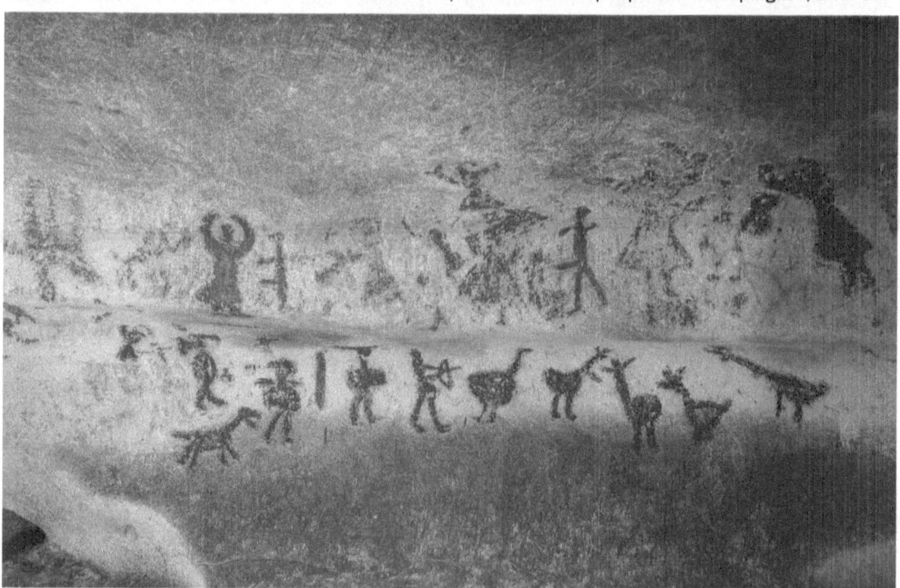

ner they burned all leftover food on their campfire as a sacrifice, facilitating peaceful sleep. The next time they ate would have been after a night's sleep. In the morning, men set up their traps and nets and they would pick fruits found on trees on their way to their hunting grounds. As they were hungry and thirsty in the morning, they consumed the fruit immediately, never bringing it back to the camp. Fruit is sweet, supplying instant energy but heavy to transport without a bag. The women, elderly people and children commenced their daily gathering activities satisfying their hunger and thirst with sweet and juicy fruits.

They also gathered vegetables and wild grains but only brown rice, oats and rye were available for them compared to the abundance of grains consumed nowadays. Other grains were rare, and only a restricted amount was gathered from them for food. Our early ancestors did not eat wheat, corn and oilseeds. Drinking animal milk was not considered, as they only hunted animals and did not breed them.

Before the heat of noon, the hunting groups and those gathering vegetables and grains went back to the camp. Water was brought by the hunters in leather carriers, as usually traps were placed near waterholes. Lunch was prepared around noon for the hungry group. They poured water in special leather containers, added wild rice, oats, rye and root vegetables if they had found any. Then stones that were heated in the fire were put into the water, boiling it quickly. Adding heated stones helped to maintain the temperature until the rice was soft and edible. The resulting mush was flavored by vegetables and basil or honey. Almonds, nuts, peas and beans were only consumed over a short period of the year when they were found in the wild. In the afternoon, men went to fetch meat while women gathered firewood. They could drink water at waterholes to soothe their thirst.

If the hunters found anything in their traps, they immediately brought it back to the camp to protect their catch from predators by the use of fire. If the traps were empty, they checked their fishing nets in streams or seas nearby. Their dinner consisted of wild meat or fish with vegetables, depending on the success of their fishing or hunting and gathering.

If no fish were caught in their nets, they attempted to harpoon some. If they still failed, they took more hazardous activities like hunting to secure their dinner. Using weapons made of sharp stones, they hunted larger birds and gathered eggs from their nests. They consumed every part of the meat of the birds including the offal.

This is how our ancestors lived day by day. Not for fun - this was their only means of survival. Their environment was wild; any careless move could expose them to predators to hunt them down. If they were unsuccessful at hunting, fishing and gathering, they ate only fruits or in some cases, anything they could find – or sometimes they went to bed hungry.

Their body make-up including their teeth, were identical to ours in the 21st century. However, excavations have proven that they were never sick, since rough conditions compelled them to have a daily eating routine. They followed it to such an extent that even if given the opportunity, they did not diverge from their eating custom. For example, if one of them hunted down a turkey in the morning, he brought it back to the camp and placed it safely next to the fire. But he went back to his usual activity and left cooking for later when the group began the usual dinner preparation activities. Our daily biorhythm developed according to these customs.

Approximately two million years ago, all human beings living on Earth, developed a dental structure identical to ours today. This indicates the absolute adaptation of humans to the consumption of cooked food. They had larger teeth and jaws in the past, which indicates the consumption of raw food. It was simultaneous with the shrinkage of the human digestive system and the substantial loss of body hair. The number of sweat glands significantly increased, empowering them with advanced thermoregulation by perspiration during great physical effort on hot African afternoons.

These transformations enabled humans to become excellent long-distance swimmers and the best long-distance runners on Earth, vital for hunting prey. For this reason, two million years ago our ancestors in Africa developed a new hunting technique helping them to gain huge amounts of red meat. They approached their prey while it rested in the afternoon heat, then they chased it relentlessly without stopping. The reason for this was to exhaust it causing a heat stroke to the animal within one or two hours. They finished it with a heavy blow to its head. Bushmen, nowadays still use this hunting tactic.

Our ancestors drifted over in small groups to the European continent until their descendants populated the whole continent, migrating to other areas and continents to populate the entire planet. Our European ancestors had no way to apply the hunting tactics described above because of the woody and bushy terrain and colder weather. Therefore, they rather hunted fowls using sharpened stone weapons, and besides fishing, hunting red meat less frequently. The resulting increase in protein intake catalyzed the development of the human brain. This means that our ancestors, until the technical revolution in recent times, had been constrained to these eating customs for almost two million years, since they could only chew cooked food.

During the course of two million years of evolution, the human body, digestive system and biorhythm have adapted completely to this pattern of eating. It is widely accepted that colds, fungal diseases, allergies, obesity, poor eyesight, diabetes, cancer and heart attacks are unfortunate but inescapable features of human life. However, these were not natural for our ancestors, whose genes we carry. It is proven by excavations that everybody, including your ancestors, had perfect vision without the need for glasses, and no such diseases at all. If they had had any kind of diseases in the wild, they could not have survived and you would not be reading these lines. Deviating from the eating customs which developed naturally over millions of years, weakens and sickens people.

By examining the daily routine of our ancestors, focusing on its core components, intense physical activity was an important part of their daily routine. Before noon they ate fruits exclusively, two or three times depending on their route to their hunting grounds. At noon, they prepared a mush containing wholegrain rice, oats, rye and vegetables. In the afternoon they could quench their thirst with spring water, before the most important meal of the day. For dinner they usually alternated roast meat with fish, together with roast and raw vegetables. Deviation from this practice was rare, occurring only in unfortunate situations, when they would eat fruits or nothing at all for the whole day. At this time, each individual was blood group O.

The first significant change in diet happened when some groups of people observed that some grains, accidentally dropped around the camp, sprouted and grew. Before long they would spread grains on purpose, in order to easily harvest them around the camp. They found out that dried grains could be stored for more than a year. Soon they learned to grow grasses with larger ears such as wheat, sunflower and corn, as they yielded much more than oats or rye. Harvesting them was likewise easier. These grains are rarely found in nature; being larger and more conspicuous and supplying plenty of food, they are often eaten unripe by birds, deer or other animals, making them barely available for our ancestors. Accordingly, our ancestors figured out that sowing them as described above supplied them with large amounts of food of this type. This is how plant-cultivating societies emerged, where the main source of food was derived from cultivated plants: vegetables, cucurbitaceous plants (such as squashes and melons), fruits, grains, wheat, rice, corn, buckwheat, oats, nuts, sunflower and other oily seeds, leguminous plants, soy, coffee and other types of beans, peas and lentils.

Approximately 20,000 years ago in Asia and the Middle East, meat came to be in short supply since hunting became hazardous due to predators such as the big cats, scorpions, venomous snakes, and other dangerous animals. For this reason, people in such areas had similar experiences to individuals today with blood group O who do not follow a conscious diet. They became weak, obese and sickly, their teeth and eyesight deteriorated, they suffered from osteoporosis, diabetes, and often died from cardiovascular diseases.

Similarly, artifacts excavated in Egypt undoubtedly indicate that as their dietary habits and customs changed due to the introduction of wheat cultivation, Egyptians in perfect health suddenly became obese. Previously unknown diseases then began to decimate the population, namely type 2 diabetes and cardiovascular diseases. Instead of obtaining their carbohydrates from fruits, brown rice or oats, they began to consume wheat. At that time there was no sugar or other harmful ingredient to blame. Only wheat appeared in their menu replacing the whole grains they had consumed before.

These factors caused the first significant genetic alteration in the history of mankind. Over a short period of time, due to a process called ultra-selection, a new group evolved, known as blood type A.

The expression "blood type" is quite misleading, as it indicates a variation concerning only the blood of humans, as it was believed at the beginning. The genes of blood group A adjusted to the habits of the plant-cultivating society. Dominant genes in blood type A overwrite the genes of blood type O. Blood type A has completely different genes to blood type O: the stomach became alkaline, not acidic, in order to digest cultivated plants instead of meat.

In a person of blood type A, the whole digestive system, musculature and temperament are adjusted to the habits of the new society. Their body is prepared to handle the excessive oil and sugar content of wheat, maize and other plants, which in blood group O individuals cause obesity, cardiovascular diseases, diabetes and joint diseases. Blood type A individuals are less effective in gaining muscular strength from animal protein; their muscles basically work by burning carbohydrates. Thus, they cannot make as swift and huge physical efforts as people with type O blood, their muscles and joints are weaker than those of blood group O. However, they have a greater talent for languages and forward thinking, and they are more resistant to infectious diseases, due to antibodies in their red blood cells.

As groups of predominantly blood type A grew, they developed settlements or towns, sharing the products of their labour. Professions such as miller, baker, carpenter, stonemason, fisherman and so on developed.

Their only source of animal protein was fish caught before noon, which they could buy and trade in early afternoon markets. Fish spoils quickly in warm-climate countries. As refrigeration was not an option for thousands of years, blood group A individuals consumed fish only on the day it was caught, until 1748 when William Cullen invented the basis of modern refrigeration.

By paying attention to the important parts of their routine, eating fruits in the morning was usually their first activity. However, by noon, as soon as the baker was ready, a large variety of whole-grain bakery products was available to them, supplemented by oily seeds such as pistachio, poppy, nuts, sunflower seed and almond. Their sweetener was honey by then. So

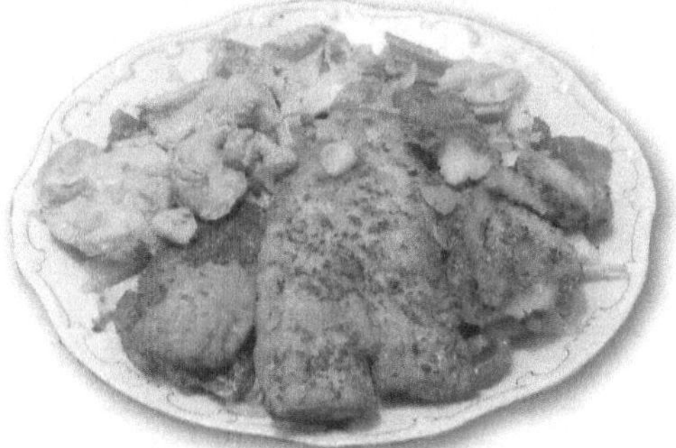

they had the opportunity to eat when they awoke or just to have a lunch around midday. Apart from fish dishes, their main protein source was leguminous plants: beans, soy, peas, lentils. By using the drying process known as desiccation, they were edible all year round.

For the main meal, they often roasted fish garnished with cultivated vegetables such as carrot, celery, beetroot, parsnip and other bulbous or root vegetables. Sometimes the fish catch would be poor, so they cooked and dined on protein-rich leguminous vegetables, usually cooked together with brown rice and other plants. They already used crockery to cook their lunches and dinners, and used a rich variety of spices, flavoring their meals as they desired. Applying these and preparing various ingredients, they could diversify their meals and flavors.

People with blood type A occasionally slaughtered some poultry wandering around their crops, but they did not hunt or breed animals. Hence milk, red meat, and offal never constituted a part of their meal. Blood group A individuals adjusted to this nutritional custom and today would probably be classed as a largely vegetarian society.

The cultivation of plants needs no huge efforts, so their daily activities were easy. Their diet, unlike that of blood group O, consisted of plants that were rarely found in nature but easily cultivated: wheat, corn, rice, beans, soy, lentils, peas, sunflower seed and nuts. Hence blood type A superseded blood type O in early agrarian societies. Subsequently, they began breeding poultry in some of these societies. For this reason, people with blood type A can easily digest poultry and eggs.

The second significant genetic alteration in human evolution occurred when, approximately ten thousand years ago in the Caucasian Steppes, people realized that by gathering herbivorous animals, such as sheep, goats and cows and leaving them in herds to graze and breed, they no longer needed to hunt in order to satisfy their hunger for meat.

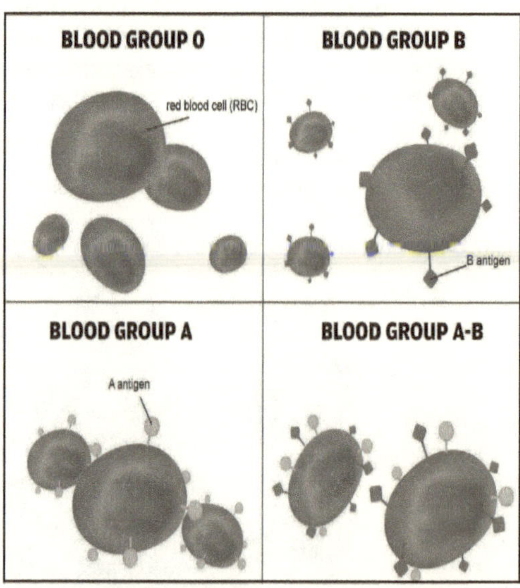

Different antibodies on the red blood cells of the four types of blood

Breeding livestock went smoothly until it was realized that some females provide consumable milk. Humans were the first living beings on Earth that drank milk after the early stage of suckling from the mother, drinking the milk of an animal, which was fresh and tasty.

Milk is essential in the first few months of a baby's life, but only the mother's breast milk. It contains special elements essential for the baby until the digestive and immune systems are well-developed, but not after. Since we only possess the required enzymes to digest lactose and milk protein in our childhood, milk after that time can cause obesity, allergies, diabetes, joint inflammation and other health problems for blood type O and A individuals in their adulthood. The digestive system senses the consumed dairy product and attempts to break down its elements, but due to the lack of the requi-

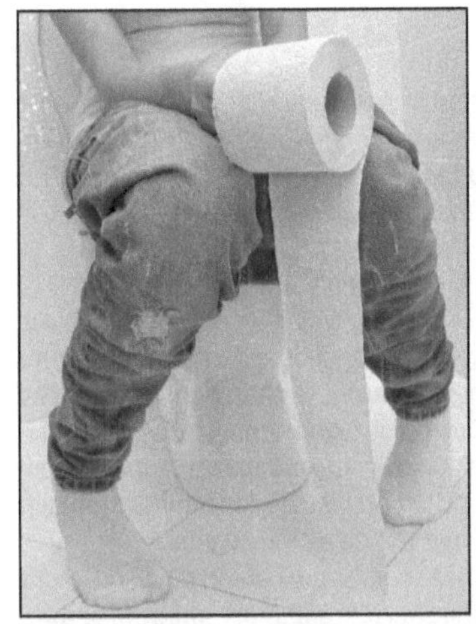

red enzymes, digestion is impossible.

Milk starts to spoil at 97°F. Having no other option, the human body's vegetative nervous system removes the infectious content from the alimentary canal in the form of diarrhea. So besides milk, other nourishing nutriments are excreted as well. Therefore, since previously consumed food does not remain in the colon for digestion and absorption, only sugar is absorbed causing obesity, diabetes and cardiovascular diseases. Valuable nutriments, as well as energy vital for digestion, are wasted due to the consumption of milk. If this occurs only occasionalyly, it is still very harmful to the body; however, blood group O and A individuals are in greater danger if they consume dairy products daily. Because these dairy consumers suffer with diarrhea only for a few days, and afterwards their excrement is not liquid any more, but it is still undigested. This is why they lose the most important nutriments from their digestive systems. This is how dairy products often cause osteoporosis for blood group O and A individuals, regardless of any calcium content, as it goes directly into the toilet.

Returning to our friends in the Caucasian Steppes, regular dairy product consumption has affected them as well and they weakened to such a level that a third type of humans emerged in the course of human evolution, a group of people with blood type B, who continue to be able to digest milk and lactose into adulthood.

Blood group B individuals lived nomadic life in tribes, wandering and pasturing their herds on the Caucasian Steppes, trading with salt, spices, jewelry, dairy products and other goods, developing great business and communication skills. Their eating custom, except for dairy and poultry consumption, was very similar to blood group O individuals. For breakfast, they ate citrus and alkaline fruits, bananas, grapes, dates, etc. For lunch, they consumed self-sown plants like those in blood group O did: rice, oats, rye and vegetables. For the evening meal, they had meat from their livestock or fish, or they obtained dinner by trading. Poultry was rarely on their menu, but dairy products were consumed massively. Although they are more tolerant to cultivated plants than blood group O individuals, these plants are still unhealthy for them. Blood type B features are determined by blood group B dominant genes, which overwrite blood type O genes.

A fourth group, blood group AB, is the result of globalization. If somebody inherits blood type A genes from one parent, and blood type B genes from the other, a new blood type emerges from the encounter of two sets of dominant genes. People with blood type AB are able to digest all kinds of food without complications. Because they came into existence by the random encounter of genes, and as technical development enabled people to move longer distances, their lifestyle will not be analyzed in this book. We could claim that their existence is an evolutionary response to their altered nutrition, permitting the digestion of each and every type of food which we can consume nowadays.

This is how the four types of humans evolved; each of them is specialized to a certain lifestyle and nutritional custom. If you are curious about your genetic ancestors' lifestyle, whose genes you have, check your blood type, and you will find the answer to the question:

„Which foods are healthy and which foods are harmful for you?"

The Operation of our Digestive System

On a fundamental level, all of the blood groups have a similar digestive system, they are only specialized to break down different foods. The first step and a precondition of healthy digestion is thorough chewing to mix food with saliva. It is essential to have healthy teeth to chew food into small pieces as this is necessary for digestion. The use of an electric blender is advised if chewing is difficult or not preferred for any reason.

Swallowing the food moves it from the mouth through the gullet to the stomach, where it is pre-digested. The digestion is controlled by the vegetative nervous system, which works automatically, similarly to the heartbeat. For this reason, our brain does not receive feedback information from the stomach. Therefore, we are inclined to believe that we have no trouble eating and mixing any kinds of foods, entrusting our stomach to digest anything. Our brain follows the process until the food is swallowed and from that point, there is no further conscious control. Appropriate digestive juices are secreted by our stomach according to the type of food we previously consumed. Stomach movements help the digestive enzymes to mix with the food, and the digestion begins.

The human digestive system basically can apply three digestive programs to break down different types of foods. Only one program can run at once. The first is the shortest and most simple program, taking the least energy from our body. This is only used by our digestive system when we consume exclusively fresh and not heat-treated fruits. If, besides fruit, any other type of food is consumed before the end of pre-digestion, even in the smallest portion such as a bite of bread or meat, the stomach switches to a heavier program.

The digestion of fruit takes 15-45 minutes. Alkaline fruits with higher sugar level, such as bananas, dates, grapes and plums stay in the stomach for the longest period of time. So, if you eat a variety of fruits, start with the alkaline fruits.

Acidic fruits, such as citrus, spend the least time in the stomach. In this case, the predigested fruit eaten on an empty stomach moves through the duodenum and the small intestine into the colon without any further digestion in 20-50 minutes. Enzymes, amino acids, vitamins and minerals essential for our health, are absorbed in the colon with the rest of the nutriments,
It is worthy to note that fruits are amongst the least calorie-rich foods as 90% of the fruits is crystal-clear water.

There are only two basic sugars in them: fructose and glucose, and their sweetness is significantly stronger and more intense than the taste of other sugars such as beet, cane and brown sugar. The molecules of these sugars consist of a combination of fructose and glucose that form longer chains in them, containing the multiplicity of calories of the two basic sugars. Natural flavorings found in fruits further increase the intense sweetness of fructose, thereby the taste of fruits is significantly sweeter than their calorie levels would indicate.

Enzymes, vitamins and amino acids contained in them are essential for our body, and they can only be absorbed from non-heat-treated fresh and ripe fruits.

Before our ancestors climbed down from the trees, fruit was their only source of carbohydrates and the main source of amino acids. These then remained the main source of carbohydrates until the development of plant-cultivating societies.

When we consume seedy fruits, such as melon or grapes, we should take care to spit out seeds as masticated seeds are digested as oily seeds, hindering the easy digestion of fruit.

Anyway, fruit only contains nutriments that can be broken down from other foodstuffs, These elements, the two basic sugars and amino acids can be used by our body in biochemical processes.

This is the reason why fruits do not need prolonged digestion. The absorption of fructose and glucose begins in the stomach, providing instant energy for the beginning of the day, instead of taking away energy for the initiation of a heavier digestive program.

Thus, if we eat exclusively fruit for breakfast, our body will have the required energy for morning detoxification. It means that the absorption and the storage of toxic compounds in fatty tissues is avoided, preventing obesity and other health problems. The morning fruit pushes the remainder of last night's dinner from the small intestine into the colon, due to its slightly acidic and fibrous composition. It clears the remainders from your intestines as a chimney sweep removes ash and soot using the brush. For this purpose, apple is the best, because of its high roughage content.

If someone follows a diet with poor fruit and fiber intake, a large amount of odorous excrement will be stuck in his or her alimentary canal, poisoning the body from inside. These sticky remainders, depending on the age of the individual, may remain there for several decades and can be a substantial quantity.

I would not like to describe it further, however, if someone starts to eat healthily after a long period of time, his or her first experiences will be unpleasant, including odorous feces. This is a good sign however, meaning that excrement that has probably been stuck to the alimentary canal for a long while is being cleansed. Meanwhile, toxins stored in tissues are likewise cleaned up, and may cause nausea.

The best method to get rid of these toxins is to eat fruit exclusively and drink water and tea for one or two days. Therefore, introducing a fruit-only day from time to time to your eating routine is very useful. This is an excellent detoxification cure, best done during summer, when ripe seasonal fruits are cheap, containing the least amount of toxin, and since our body needs hydration in the hot weather, fruit consumption avoids high calorie intake. In addition, fruit digestion requires the least energy and causes the least internal heat generation, helping us to endure the heat.

The second program which our stomach and digestive system can launch is activated upon the consumption of complex carbohydrates. These carbohydrates are found in foods prepared from plants excluding fruits and vegetables. This includes all grains: rice, rye, oats, barley, wheat, corn; leguminous plants: beans, lentils and peas; oily seeds: almond, sunflower seeds, nuts and poppy seeds; fruit and vegetable seeds such as pumpkin, apricot, grape and melon seeds. Different complex carbohydrates can be predigested in the stomach with the same alkaline enzymes.

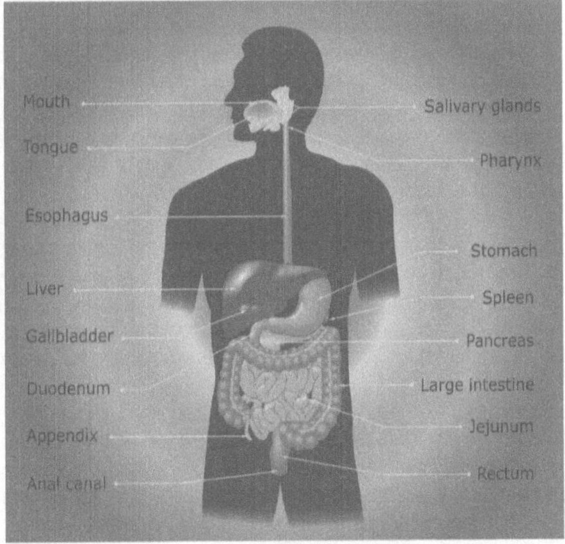

Although potato is a vegetable, because of its high content of starch, it belongs to the complex carbohydrates. Besides these foods, all types of vegetables are digested perfectly by this second program. It lasts for three hours in the stomach, an additional one or two hours in the small intestine and ends in the colon. During this process, the digestive system breaks down vegetable protein to amino acids, and starch and complex carbohydrates to glucose and fructose, using alkaline digestive enzymes.

The second program needs much more energy than the first, but still a moderate amount. Our ancestors digested their vegan lunch with this program for two million years, thus around mid-afternoon, already they were full of energy to acquire meat for dinner. Therefore, according to our natural daily biorhythm, in the late afternoon hours, (the time when our ancestors hunted), we are able to make the greatest physical effort.

The third program which our stomach and digestive system can launch, digests meat and other animal proteins. It is longer, more complex, and uses more energy than the second program, running about four hours in the stomach and 2-3 hours in the small intestine, ending in the colon. According to the type of meat or fish we consume, different types of specific acidic digestive enzymes are produced in our stomach, pancreas and small intestine in order to disintegrate various protein chains. So, different acidic enzymes are needed to break down different kinds of fish, poultry or meat of mammals to amino acids. For this reason, only one type of meat or fish is digestible by our digestive system at a time, thus different types of meat or fish should be eaten separately on different days. So for dinner you should consume the meat and offal of only one species of animal with vegetables.

For example, choosing duck for dinner, we can have duck leg, duck liver, duck heart, duck gizzard, eggs, but leave chicken for another day. If we have hake fish for dinner, it is best to have hake and its parts exclusively. The following day, for instance, we could eat beef, then the next day only herring, the day after only turkey and eggs, afterwards only tuna fish and so on. Adding vegetables to meat and fish dishes is strongly recommended, as they are essential for the digestion of animal protein. Eggs and dairy products are built from more simple proteins, hence easily digested with fish and poultry. However, be aware that milk and mammal meat are not digestible together. Vegetables are broken down by both acidic and alkaline digestive enzymes. Vegetable fiber carries bacteria which are essential for meat digestion, these reproduce naturally as they pass through the gut and the colon. Pay attention to distinguishing vegetables from fruit and leguminous plants! If we appropriately pair protein from animals and vegetables, then after four hours, the content of the stomach moves through the duodenum to the small intestine, where, based on the type of proteins consumed, it is mixed with bile and other digestive enzymes. Digestion continues in the small intestine for another three hours, then ends in the colon, where the amino acids derived from proteins are absorbed, constituting the materials that our body uses during deep sleep to rebuild our cells and tissues.

Due to our natural biorhythm, our deep sleep usually takes place between 2am and 5am. During this process, our body is regenerated, muscles are built, injuries are healed, and children grow. For this reason, vast amounts of amino acids are needed for this process, as our body builds its proteins from them.

If we consume our dinner as our ancestors did for two million years, i.e. eating meat and vegetables around 7-8 pm, then the consumed food spends 4 hours in our stomach and 3 hours in our small intestine, arriving to our colon around 2-3 am. There, besides further digestion, proteins in the form of amino acids are absorbed, synchronized to the peak demand for them.

So, our blood and lymphatic system will be full of proteins, amino acids and lipids essential for our cells, awaiting only two other things. The first is the glucose or fructose for protein synthesis, lipogenesis and the rebuilding of our ATP supply.

The second is the opening of our cell membranes to let these materials enter into the cells. Both of these processes are continued by the wholegrain complex carbohydrates consumed for lunch and finished by the effect of fruits consumed for breakfast. Glucose and fructose are immediately absorbed in the stomach.

Consequently, a hormone called insulin, stored in the pancreas, is infiltrated into the blood circulation. Connecting to specific cell receptors, insulin opens up cell membranes, enabling the inflow of glucose, fructose, amino acids, ATP, lipids, and K-ions into the cells.
The insulin increases glycogen synthesis, lipogenesis, glycogenolysis, protein synthesis, and the concentration of growth hormones in numerous cells. Inside the cells, it increases growth and the synthesis of proteins and nucleic acids.

Briefly, fruit consumed in the morning activates the body by causing an insulin injection immediately into the blood circulation. The glucose, amino acids, and enzymes, aided by vitamins, complete their effects reacting to the complex working of insulin, rapidly empowering us to use great physical effort as our cells are filled with energy. It seems that insulin in the morning originally functioned as an alert mechanism. Reacting to fruit intake, insulin activates our cells in the morning. The idleness overnight is over - energize yourself, activity is coming!

This system works perfectly, as easy digestion needs only a small amount of energy for a short period of time. Our body is capable of using energy for other activities, such as physical exercise, detoxification, fat-burning and thinking. For this reason, if our body receives appropriate meals at the right time, our hunger is satisfied with a smaller intake of food. Furthermore, healthy digestion produces significantly less toxins, optimizing the workings of our body by numerous methods.
Keeping up with this diet, our ageing slows down as our cells receive proper nutriments at the time when they are needed, and due to a less toxic environment, our cells will live longer together with us. Our digestive system can run these three digestive programs discussed above.
What happens when we deviate from our ancestors' patterns, and consume complex carbohydrates with animal protein? If, for instance, we eat one or two salami sandwiches with a peach, our stomach, sensing the presence of consumed food, applies the second program without other options, predigesting the complex carbohydrates. Alkaline digestive juices soak the bread, as well as the meat, in vain. For this reason, our stomach needs to produce twice as much alkaline digestive juice as normally needed.

Using the second program, our stomach struggles to digest twice the amount of food as it should do otherwise. Meanwhile, the meat remains undigested in the 97°F alkaline fluids, hence it starts to spoil.

After three hours, the bread would normally have been digested and moved forward, however, sensing the undigested meat, everything stays in the stomach. Our digestive system, unlike our brains, cannot select foods, thus it applies the third acidic program to predigest the remaining meat. However, in order to start with the acidic pre-digestion, the stomach needs to neutralize its existing alkaline contents; therefore it requires twice the amount of acidic juices normally needed to digest meat. Then the stomach becomes neutral and continues to produce twice the amount of acidic juices as normally needed, to make its climate acidic for the digestion of the meat, even though the predigested bread should not be soaked in acidic fluids. Our stomach needs approximately an hour to turn its climate from alkaline to acidic. This way, after four hours waiting, the pre-digestion of slightly rotten meat is about to begin. For this, four times the amount of acidic digestive juices and the multiplicity of energy are needed as in the case of consuming exclusively meat and vegetables.

Have you ever felt acid in your throat? Of course, our stomach still needs to struggle with twice as much food, and after a further four hours, when the meat is also predigested and substances from the stomach are moving through the duodenum to the small intestine, the digestive system needs twice as much gall to digest the meat in the small intestine, requiring another three hours.

This type of inefficient digestion absorbs 80% of our body's potential energy level for 11 hours. It takes a vast amount of energy from our life-force, in vain. This means that the consumed food needs 11 hours to arrive into the colon, where proper absorption starts. This is way too long.

The peach, requiring no disintegration for digestion, would normally have arrived in the colon in 40 minutes. Instead, it was soaked for 11 hours along with the bread and the meat, in 97°F alkaline fluids, then in acidic fluids, rotting in vain. Valuable vitamins and enzymes were wasted. Similarly, the digestion of bread lasted for 11 hours, instead of 4-5 hours. At least it does not have many nutrients to lose, nonetheless it has spoiled slightly. Similarly, the meat spoiled, having to sit in the digestive system for 11 hours at 97°F.

Fortunately, eggs and milk were not consumed in this example. This type of digestion is stressful for the body, taking away our life energy, sending spoiled foods into our colon after half a day of struggle, creating a vast amount of toxins. If our brain were able to receive feedback from this process, everyone would certainly eat complex carbohydrates with animal proteins only once in their lifetime, never again. As there is no feedback of this type, we need to be conscious and careful about healthy nutrition. We should choose proper meals, appropriately timed.

Utilizing our increased intellect, we have conquered nature. Thanks to advanced technology, we have a wide range of possibilities to shape our life. Thanks to global trade, the canned food industry and the invention of the refrigerator - contrary to our ancestors - we can consume any otherwise perishable foodstuff at any time of the day.

This is the time to realize that, although we have conquered nature, we need to control ourselves. Systematic diets ought to be introduced in order to regain the strength and health which our ancestors possessed, and which helped humans to become the superior predators on Earth.

Please note that there are certain vitamin D compounds essential for our body which cannot be obtained from natural food. They only synthesize in our body as a result of sunshine. These vitamin D compounds are essential for protection against cancer as well as for bone building. Thus, don't worry about going out in the sunshine, only repeated serious sunburn causes skin cancer. However, it is important to be careful with sunbathing to prevent unpleasant and painful sunburn.

The Principle of Regularity

First, we investigated what our ancestors ate at different parts of the day through almost the last two million years. Then we inspected the ideal working of our digestive system. Thus, we have discovered in two ways, the diet we need to follow if we wish to live without diseases, obesity, in great comfort, and as long as it is encoded in your genetics. This can last for 120 years or even longer!

The Diet for Blood Type O or B

The recommended diet (assuming you wake up at 6.15 am for example) is as follows:

Breakfast:	• *Around 6.30 am, 1 kg/2lb 3oz fruit*
	• *Around 8 am, 1 kg/2lb 3oz fruit*
	• *Around 9.30 am, 1 kg/2lb 3oz fruit*
Lunch:	• *Around 12 pm, vegan lunch made of 30-40 dag of dried whole grain complex carbohydrates with vegetables*
	• *Around 5 pm, 1.5-2 l/,6-3,5pt fluid (tea and/or still mineral water)*
Dinner:	• *Around 7 pm, dinner made 30-50 dag of animal protein and 60-70 dag of vegetables*

The Diet for Blood Type A or AB

If you feel your body needs more main meals, try to have:

Breakfast:	• *Around 6.30 am, 1 kg/2lb 3oz fruit*
	• *Around 8 am, light vegan breakfast with complex carbohydrates*
	• *Around 11 am, 1 l/1,7pt fluid(tea and/or still mineral water)*
Lunch:	• *Around 12 pm, vegan lunch*
	• *Around 5 pm, 1 l/1,7pt fluid (tea and/or still mineral water)*
Dinner:	• *Around 7 pm, dinner with high protein intake*

You should not drink anything one hour before eating or while you are eating, and for 2-3 hours after eating, since digestive juices diluted by water are not as effective as when they are at 100% concentration. Your stomach has a finite capacity, so you should satisfy your appetite with nutrients instead of water, otherwise you will not be well-nourished and able to keep to this diet system. Your diet and foodstuffs should be well aligned to your blood type! You can have neutral foods from time to time but try to avoid harmful foodstuffs and artificial additives. Use only iodinated sea salt, never artificial products!

Consume 1-2 cloves of garlic every day, but never more! Cutting a couple of cloves of garlic into salads prepared for dinner is the best way for this. Thus, your daily intake is covered, it flavors the salad, and the smell is not unpleasant during the day. Dairy products used for dressings ease the smell of garlic. If possible, always use new garlic as well as purple and red onion.

Our ancestors, before the invention of cutlery, ate poultry and fish containing tiny bones and fishbone, and eggs with shell. When we consume these kinds of foods, we should rather use a complex bone-building supplement that contains calcium and magnesium. Although people tend to prefer foods they like, you should consciously eat foods suitable for your blood type, as they are the only proper nutriment for you.

Foods unsuitable for your blood type are useless for you, even if you have a vast amount of them. Your appetite will never be satisfied since they lack the nutrients your body starves for. Thus, you only consume a huge amount of unnecessary calories by them that cause obesity amongst other health-related problems.

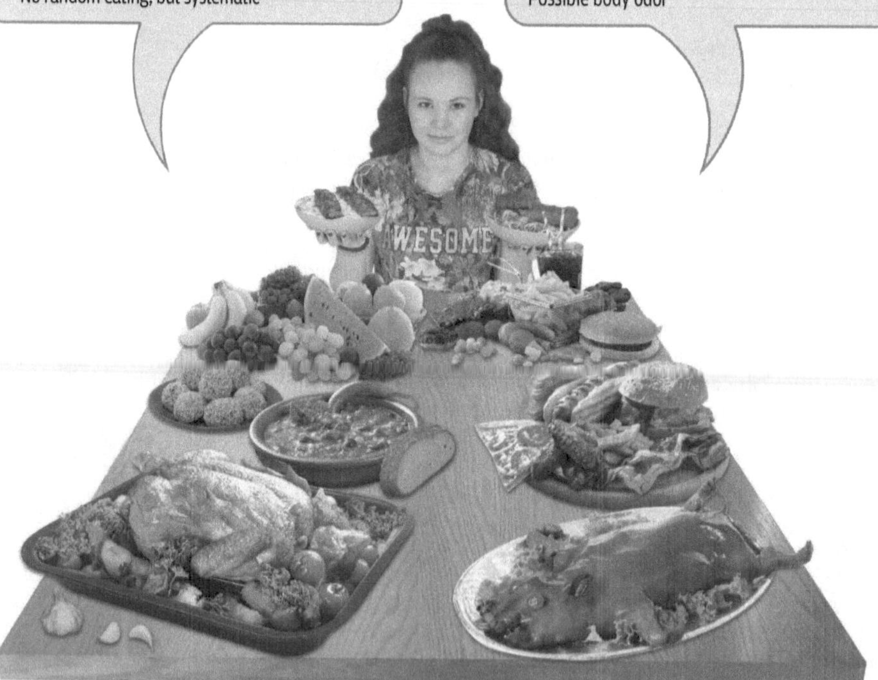

Please read on exclusively the chapter for the type of your blood.

Blood Group O

People with type O blood carry the genes of our hunter-gatherer ancestors, who became the most skilled predators on Earth. You are strong, great in combat and have excellent leadership skills. Also, you have a good sense of space and direction. The most suitable sports for you are martial arts and sports that demand great physical strength, as your body requires intense physical activities.

Your strength and stamina are most dependent on your diet. You should eat fresh, ripe, and alkaline fruits for breakfast such as bananas, grapes, dates, plums, apples, and pears. This is the only blood group which utilizes tomatoes well. Your body does not tolerate dairy products, vegetable oils, sugars, and cultivated plants such as wheat, corn, sunflower seeds and nuts, even in small quantities. These foods can cause obesity, allergies, diabetes, joint inflammations, and cardiovascular diseases in you, thus, you should completely exclude these nutrients from your diet.

You can use sour yogurt to prepare dressing for the salad of diner, it has a sour flavor as it is lactose-free. Your lunch should include self-sown grains such as brown rice, oats, and rye, supplemented by vegetables, possibly leguminous plants, almonds, walnuts and honey.

Tea, especially green tea but also black tea, has a refreshing and stimulating effect on you, so does cocoa; however, coffee is harmful for you since it expels your red blood cells, so drink strong teas instead. If you are used to drinking coffee, or addicted to it, green tea prepared from 3-4 teabags can be a great substitute for it.

Your evening meals should alternately consist of fish and poultry or red meat, garnished with vegetables. If you are of African ancestry, eat more red meat and less poultry. Be aware of your calcium and magnesium intake, essential for your bones, as your body cannot extract these minerals from any natural sources, other than bones and egg shells.

If you eat eggs, fish, or poultry for dinner, take 500-800 mg calcium (Ca) and 200- 300 mg magnesium (Mg) before your meal. The best way is to take a complex bone-building supplement, as bone-building further requires zinc (Zn), manganese (Mn), and other macroelements.

In order to absorb these minerals, your body needs vitamin D3 and K1, which are found in fish, eggs, and animal offal. The quality of your sleep improves if your body gets these indispensable minerals. Your stomach is acidic because your body needs high-cholesterol foods: liver, heart and other offal, eggs, and red meat. Your body is tolerant of animal fats, but it is better to consume them moderately. Eating offal should likewise be constrained. For example, if you have half a chicken for dinner, your corresponding offal consumption should be proportional, e.g. half the liver, half the gizzard and only half the heart, or just a little more.

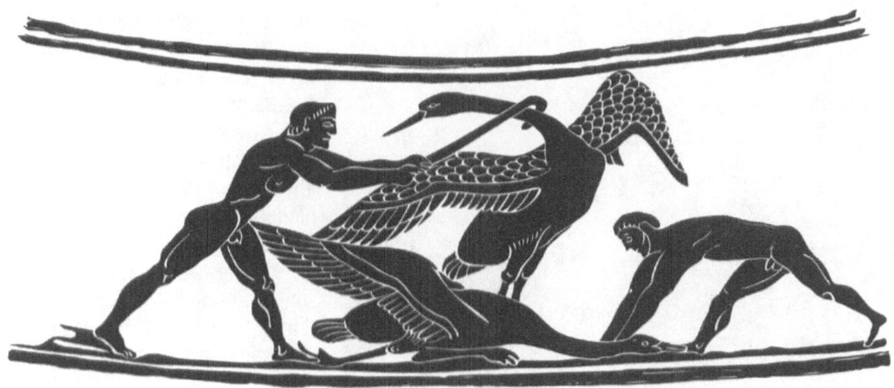

The herb basil has a healthy effect on you and it adds flavor to salads as well. If you are not concerned about gaining a little weight, consuming some nuts like almonds and pumpkin seeds will not harm you. It is good to note that more than half of the people who suffer of type 2 diabetes, are usually blood group O, and suffer with insulin resistance, caused by a deficiency of the mineral chromium.

For this reason, take a note of foods with the highest chromium content: banana, apple, blood orange, sour cherry, chicken, and broccoli.

Physicians claim that people with diabetes can safely consume fructose and glucose, since the liver absorbs these sugars from the blood without insulin medication if there is an adequate amount. In fact, diabetics should eat fruit as it can halve the number of diabetic cases by resolving chromium deficiency, and also adds enzymes, vitamins, and amino acids to the digestive system which satisfy hunger, thus preventing the excessive consumption of other high calorie foods.

Although fruits are sweet, their calorie content is low, as 90% of fruit is water. Natural sweeteners are excellent in flavoring your foods. Stevia is the best, as it is completely natural and contains 0 calories. Use honey from time to time, but a maximum of two tablespoons a day.

Individuals with blood group O who consume carbohydrates from wheat often suffer from diabetes, regardless of whether these wheats are durum or whole-grain or what is made of them (bread, rolls, scones, spaghetti or pizza) since wheat only contains elements that are useless and harmful for people of that blood group. For this reason, you will remain hungry no matter how much carbohydrate you have eaten. In addition, wheat gives you a large amount of unnecessary sugars. 100% of the wheat disintegrates in your saliva into sugars in only a couple of minutes. It is more difficult to consume the same amount of sugar in the form of pure sugars than bread, as sugars have a strong taste while bread is comparatively tasteless.

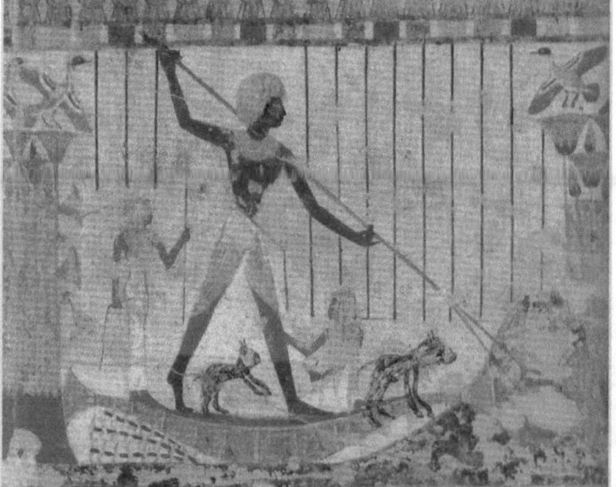

Other foodstuffs that catalyze diabetes are milk and dairy products and pork (which is strongly acidifying). These have an acidifying effect due to milk sugars and lectins. The surplus sugar is stored in the liver and fatty tissues, usually accumulated in our body until we are 35-45 years old. When these tissues are full up and our body cannot store the sugar surplus any more, insulin resistance and diabetes begin. It's recommended that every now and then - especially during the summer fruit season - you skip lunch and eat fruits during the day, which helps to endure thirst and heat.

One Week Sample Diet for Blood Group O

Sunday

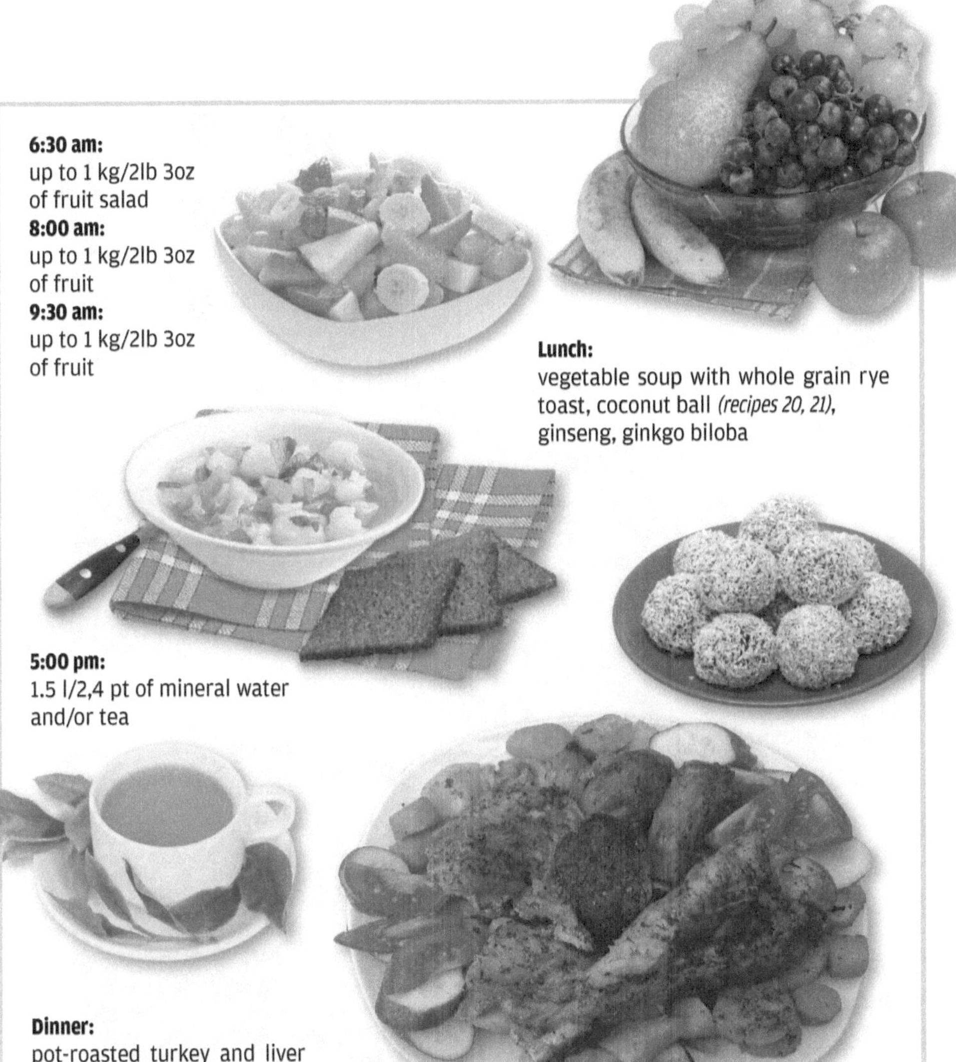

6:30 am:
up to 1 kg/2lb 3oz
of fruit salad
8:00 am:
up to 1 kg/2lb 3oz
of fruit
9:30 am:
up to 1 kg/2lb 3oz
of fruit

Lunch:
vegetable soup with whole grain rye
toast, coconut ball *(recipes 20, 21)*,
ginseng, ginkgo biloba

5:00 pm:
1.5 l/2,4 pt of mineral water
and/or tea

Dinner:
pot-roasted turkey and liver
with vegetables
(recipes 14), Ca, Mg

Blood Group O

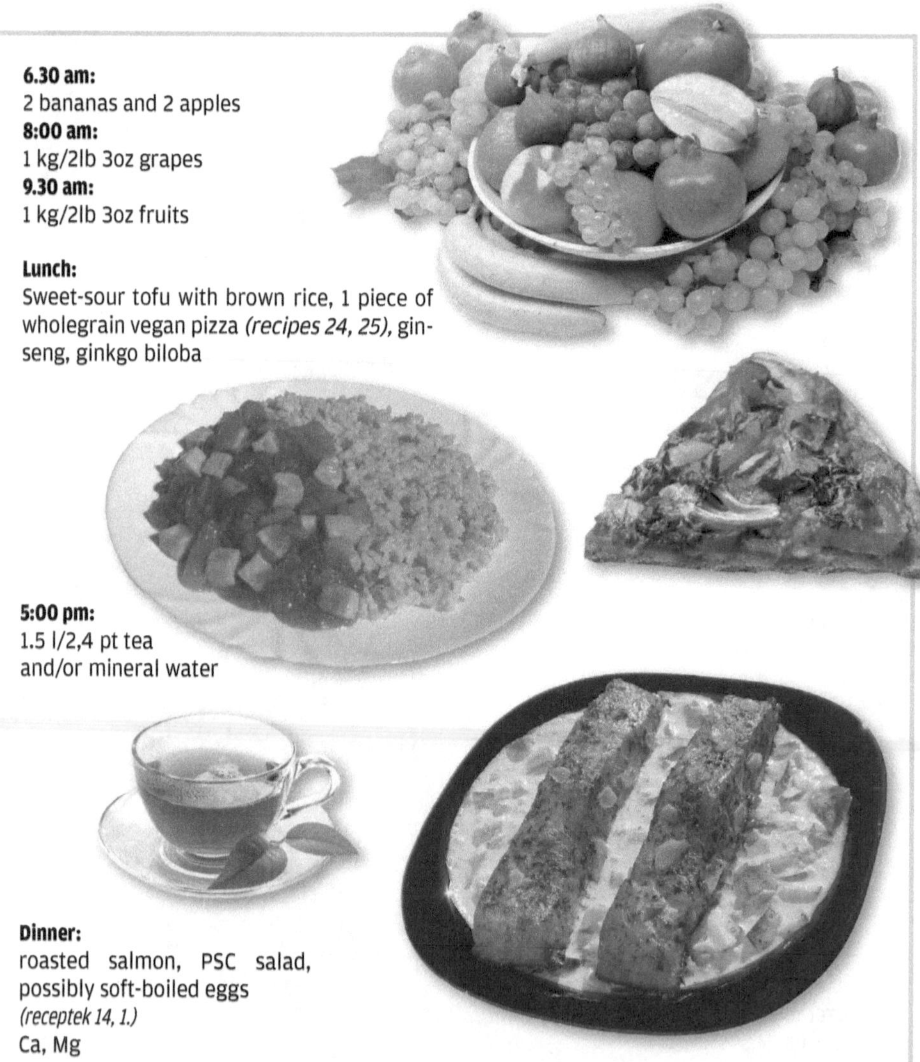

6.30 am:
2 bananas and 2 apples
8:00 am:
1 kg/2lb 3oz grapes
9.30 am:
1 kg/2lb 3oz fruits

Lunch:
Sweet-sour tofu with brown rice, 1 piece of wholegrain vegan pizza *(recipes 24, 25)*, ginseng, ginkgo biloba

5:00 pm:
1.5 l/2,4 pt tea
and/or mineral water

Dinner:
roasted salmon, PSC salad, possibly soft-boiled eggs
(receptek 14, 1.)
Ca, Mg

Blood Group 0

Tuesday

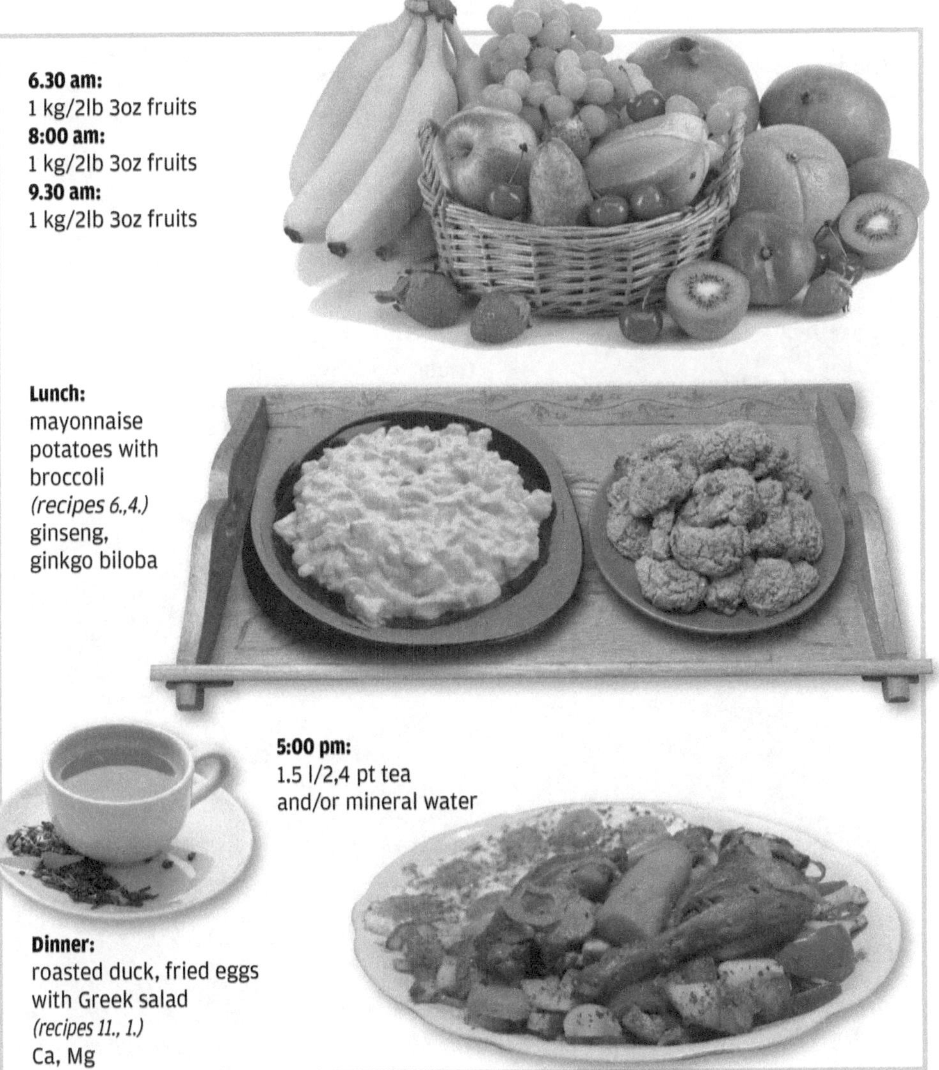

6.30 am:
1 kg/2lb 3oz fruits
8:00 am:
1 kg/2lb 3oz fruits
9.30 am:
1 kg/2lb 3oz fruits

Lunch:
mayonnaise
potatoes with
broccoli
(recipes 6.,4.)
ginseng,
ginkgo biloba

5:00 pm:
1.5 l/2,4 pt tea
and/or mineral water

Dinner:
roasted duck, fried eggs
with Greek salad
(recipes 11., 1.)
Ca, Mg

Blood Group O

6.30 am:
1 kg/2lb 3oz fruits
8:00 am:
1 kg/2lb 3oz fruits
9.30 am:
1 kg/2lb 3oz fruits

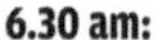

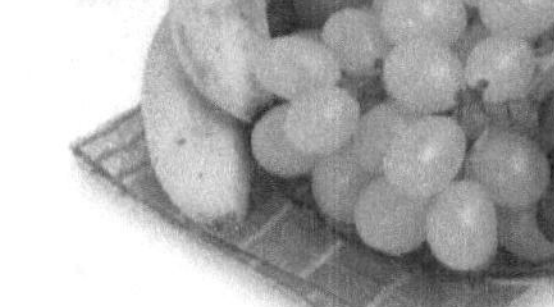

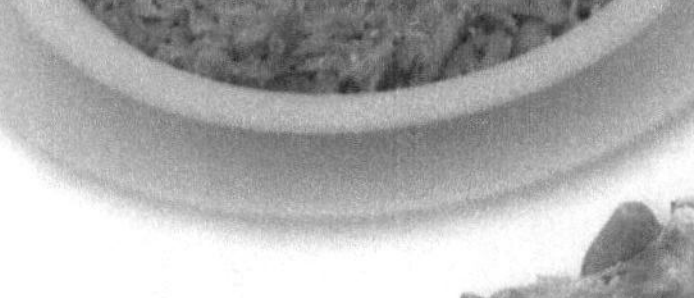

Lunch:
spaghetti Bolognese, (vegan, made of rice pasta), pancakes with seed-shake, vegetable shake *(recipes 29., 22., 3.)*

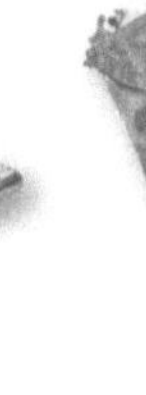

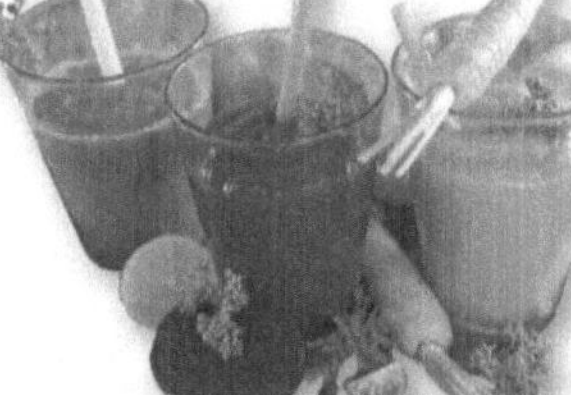

5:00 pm:
1.5 l/2,4 pt tea
and/or mineral water

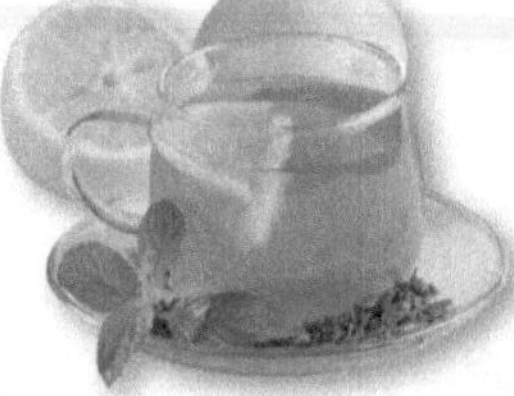

Dinner:
Agard-style fish soup – suitable for all blood types) *(recipes 16.)*
Ca, Mg

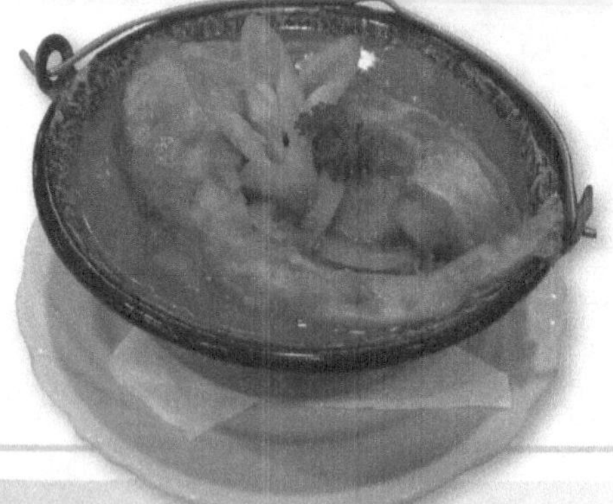

Blood Group O

Thursday

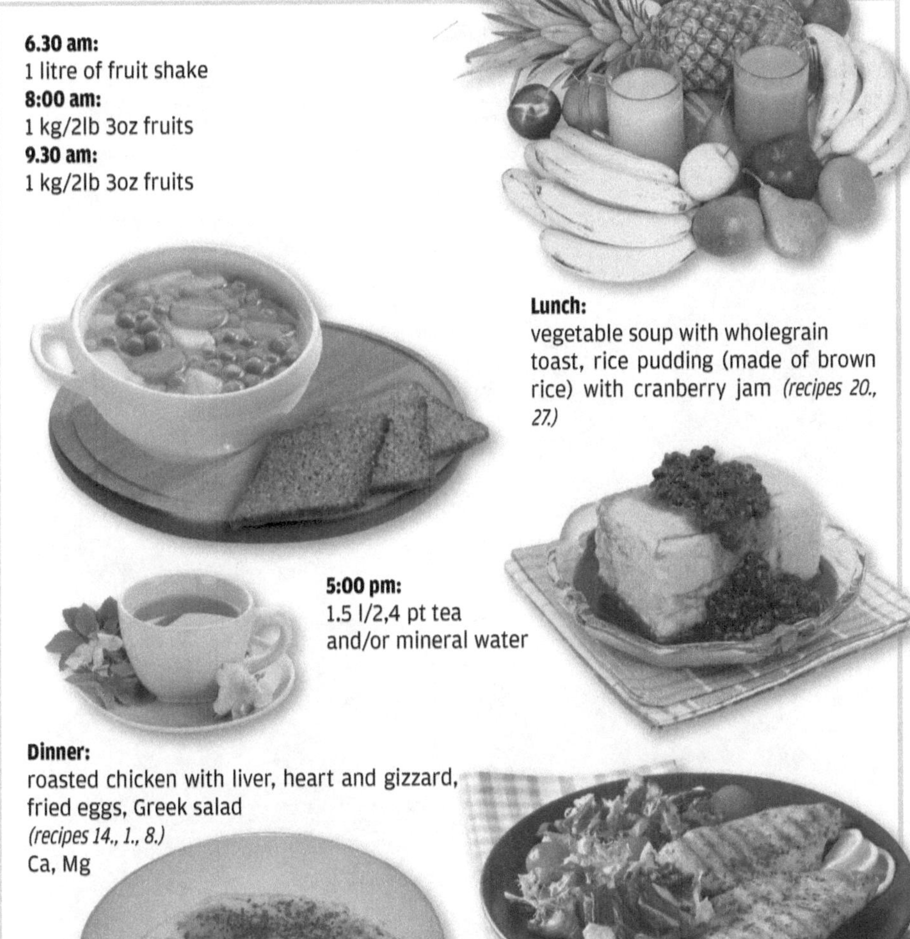

6.30 am:
1 litre of fruit shake
8:00 am:
1 kg/2lb 3oz fruits
9.30 am:
1 kg/2lb 3oz fruits

Lunch:
vegetable soup with wholegrain toast, rice pudding (made of brown rice) with cranberry jam *(recipes 20., 27.)*

5:00 pm:
1.5 l/2,4 pt tea
and/or mineral water

Dinner:
roasted chicken with liver, heart and gizzard, fried eggs, Greek salad
(recipes 14., 1., 8.)
Ca, Mg

Friday

6.30 am:
1 kg/2lb 3oz fruits
8:00 am:
1 kg/2lb 3oz fruits
9.30 am:
1 kg/2lb 3oz fruits

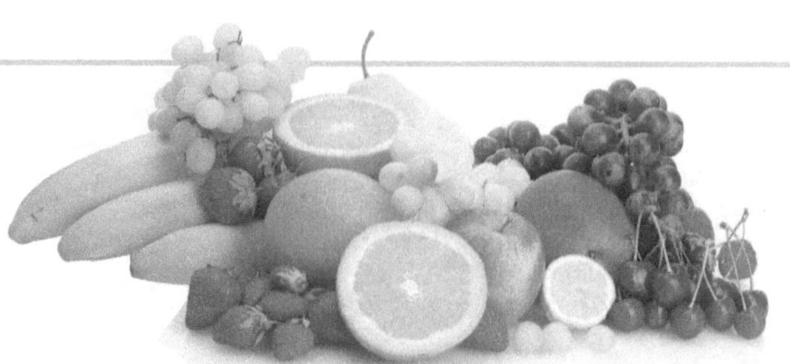

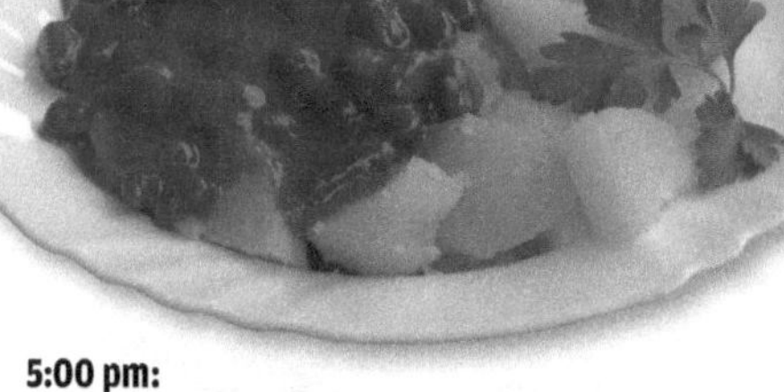

Lunch: boiled potatoes with chili beans, whole-grain rye toast, coconut balls *(recipes 7., 17., 21.)*
ginseng, ginkgo biloba

5:00 pm:
1.5 l/2,4 pt tea and/or mineral water

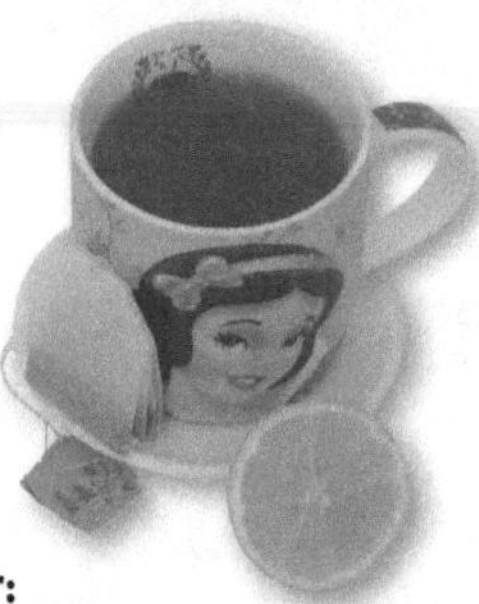

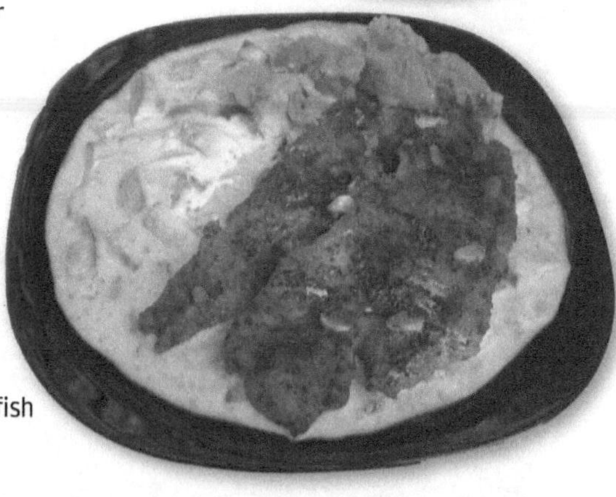

Dinner:
roasted cod fish and canned cod fish liver, PSC salad *(recipes 9., 1.)*
Ca, Mg

Blood Group O

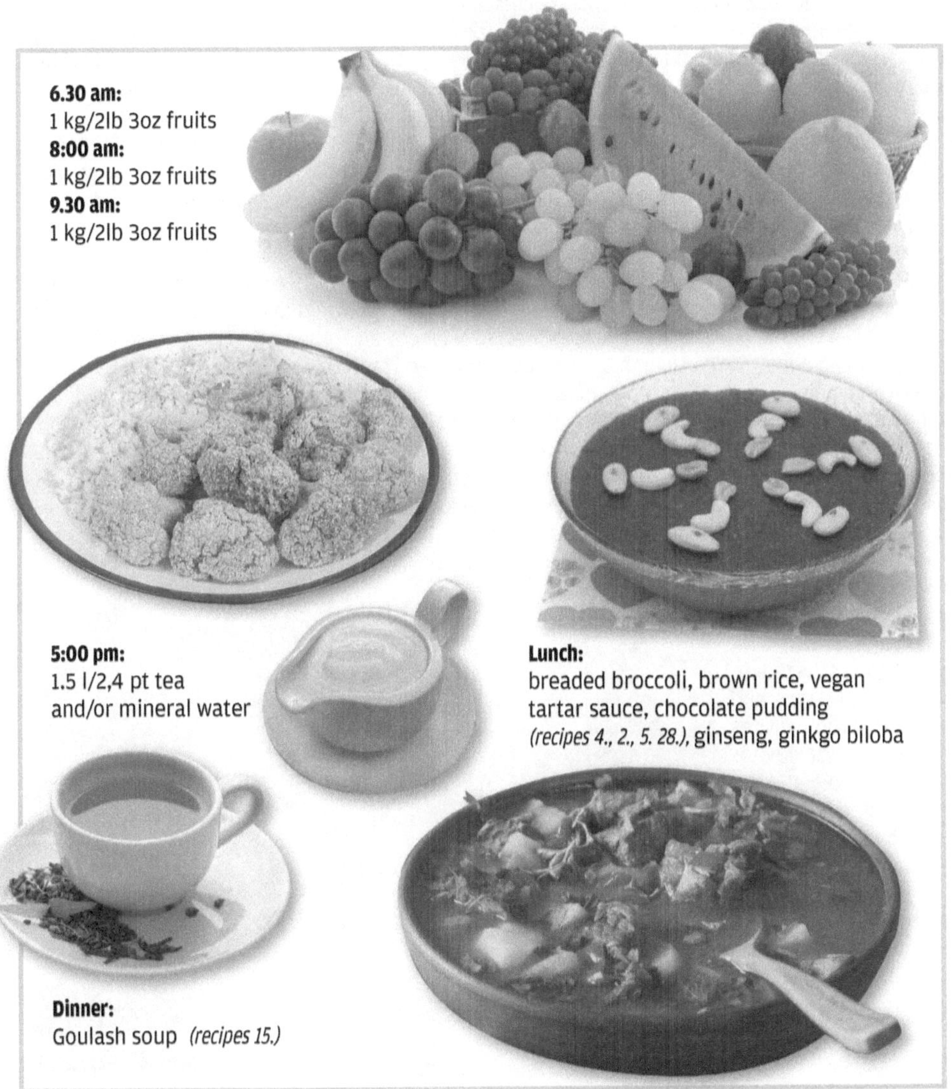

6.30 am:
1 kg/2lb 3oz fruits
8:00 am:
1 kg/2lb 3oz fruits
9.30 am:
1 kg/2lb 3oz fruits

5:00 pm:
1.5 l/2,4 pt tea
and/or mineral water

Lunch:
breaded broccoli, brown rice, vegan
tartar sauce, chocolate pudding
(recipes 4., 2., 5. 28.), ginseng, ginkgo biloba

Dinner:
Goulash soup *(recipes 15.)*

Blood Group A

People with type A blood carry the dominant genetics of our agricultural ancestors, who gave up hunting and gathering migrated to towns and began cultivating and harvesting plants, establishing the foundations of our modern societies.

You are a social person with talent for languages and forward thinking. Sports that demand less intense physical activities are suitable for you, such as yoga, tai-chi, sailing, or hiking. Your stomach is alkaline, specialized to digest cultivated plants: beans, peas, lentils, wheat, corn, barley, buckwheat, and oily seeds such as sunflower seed, poppy, nuts, and cocoa. Besides them, consumption of plants, that are also found in the wild, are likewise healthy for you such as brown rice, oats, rye and potatoes. However, your body is intolerant of cholesterol. For this reason, you should avoid eating liver, hearth, read meat especially pork, and animal fat. They may cause obesity, cancer, allergy, and bile diseases for you, and affect negatively your wellbeing due to toxins and cholesterol in them. Nowadays, consuming octopi, calamari, crabs, and shellfish is discouraged due to their high toxin levels. Tomatoes contain a type of lectin that is harmful for you, thus you should eat peppers instead. Your body tolerates vegetable oils well, but you need the amino acids, minerals, enzymes, and vitamins found in oily seeds, not the oil. Virgin olive oil is recommended for frying since it does not transform into trans-fat by heating, unlike other vegetable oils. For you fish is the best source of protein, essential amino acids, and fat-soluble vitamins. Your body is not prepared to handle toxins; hence nowadays you are subject to cancer. In your case, an increased awareness is necessary to avoid additives contained in processed and preserved foods as well as artificial colorings, sweeteners, and other preservatives. Both natural sweeteners and honey are consumable, even sugar is allowed for flavoring. Stevia is the best sweetener as it is completely natural and contains 0 calorie. You should rather have organic foods if possible!

Coffee is a favorable stimulant for you, but only brewed coffee. Instant coffees are probably very carcinogenic due to technologies used for their preparation. Be careful not to burn your food, as burned food increases the probability of cancer. If you smoke, you had better give it up as soon as possible. Although dairy products are not as harmful for you as for people with type 0 blood, avoiding them is recommended. Acidic fruits such as kiwi, peach, cherry, pineapple, citrus fruits, apple, avocado and melons are advantageous for you. Alternating fish and vegetables with beans (or other leguminous plants) and complex carbohydrates is the healthiest way for you to have diner. Also, have some poultry with vegetables from time to time. If you wish, you may alternate fish with poultry, garnished with vegetables to taste.

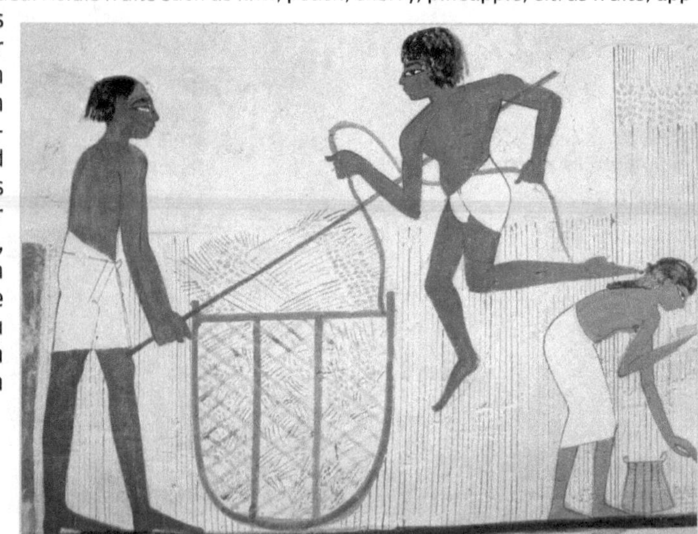

One Week Sample Diet for Blood Group A

Sunday

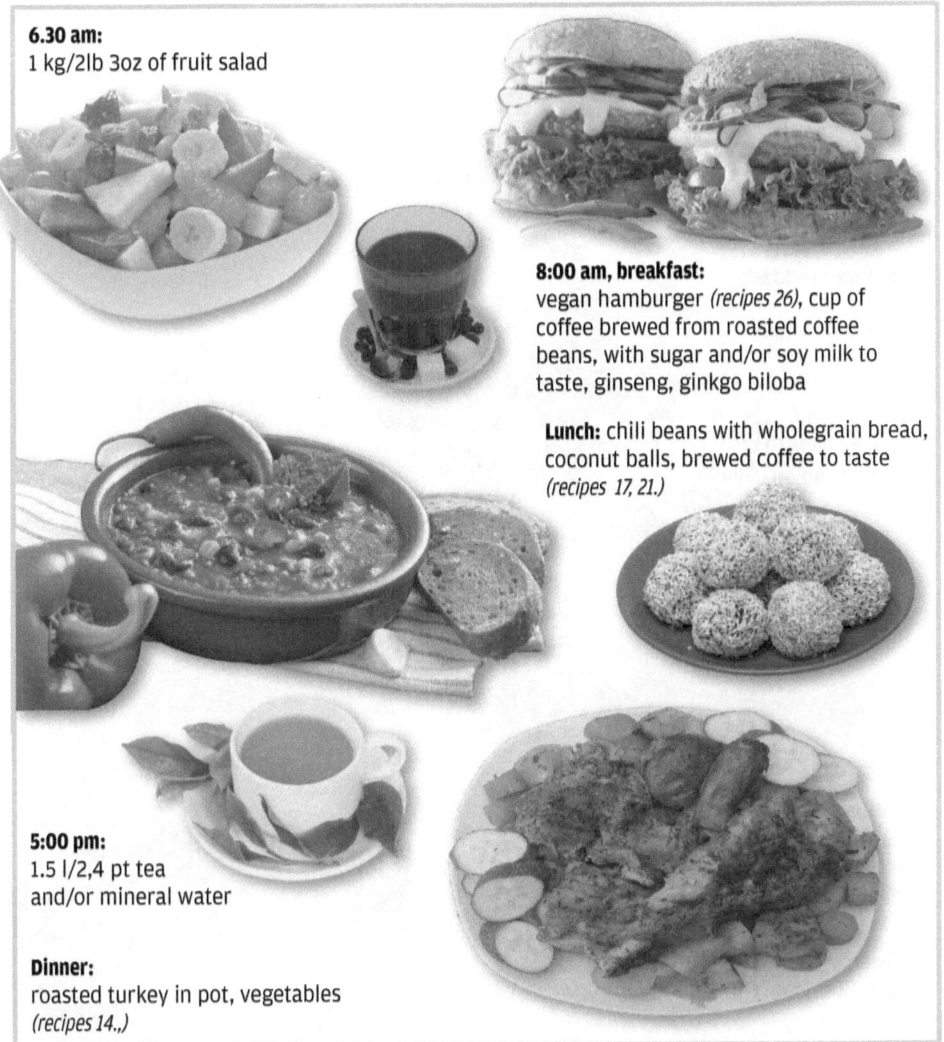

6.30 am:
1 kg/2lb 3oz of fruit salad

8:00 am, breakfast:
vegan hamburger *(recipes 26)*, cup of coffee brewed from roasted coffee beans, with sugar and/or soy milk to taste, ginseng, ginkgo biloba

Lunch: chili beans with wholegrain bread, coconut balls, brewed coffee to taste *(recipes 17, 21.)*

5:00 pm:
1.5 l/2,4 pt tea and/or mineral water

Dinner:
roasted turkey in pot, vegetables
(recipes 14.,)

Blood Group A

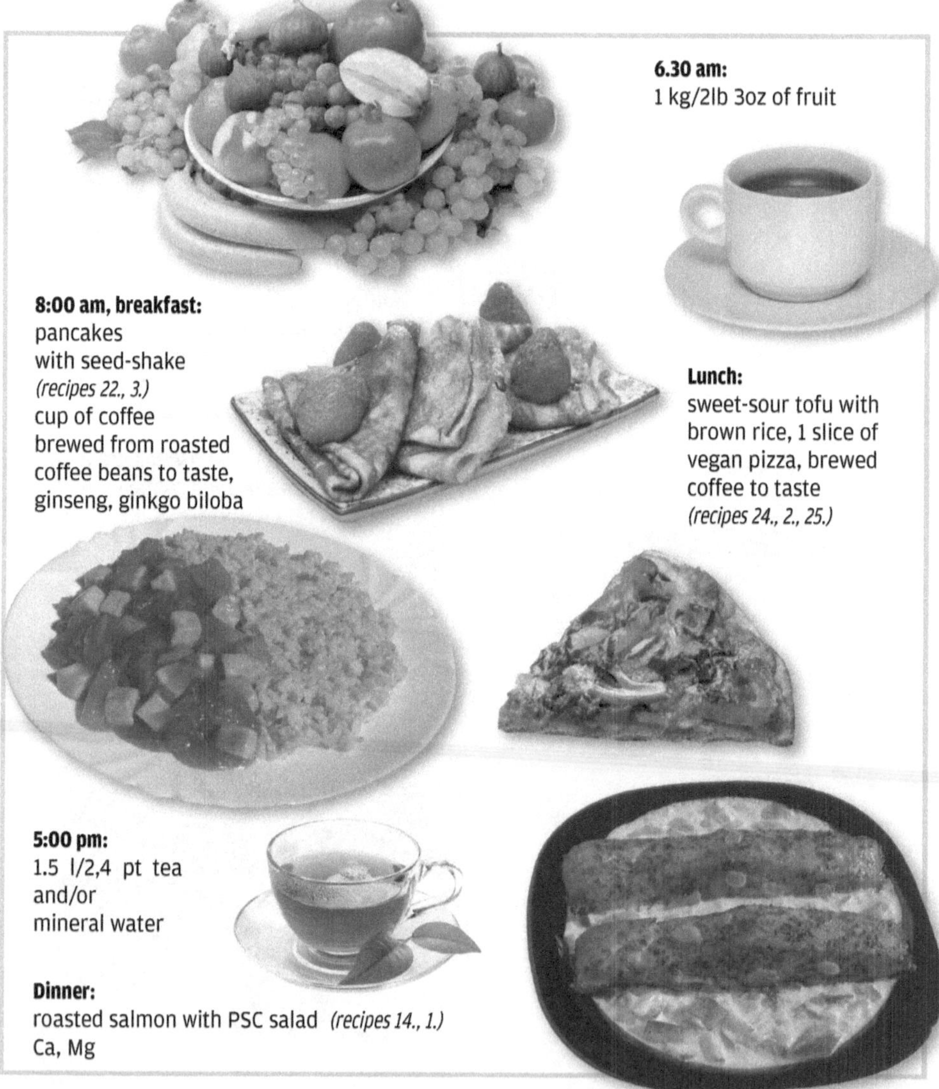

6.30 am:
1 kg/2lb 3oz of fruit

8:00 am, breakfast:
pancakes
with seed-shake
(recipes 22., 3.)
cup of coffee
brewed from roasted
coffee beans to taste,
ginseng, ginkgo biloba

Lunch:
sweet-sour tofu with
brown rice, 1 slice of
vegan pizza, brewed
coffee to taste
(recipes 24., 2., 25.)

5:00 pm:
1.5 l/2,4 pt tea
and/or
mineral water

Dinner:
roasted salmon with PSC salad *(recipes 14., 1.)*
Ca, Mg

Tuesday

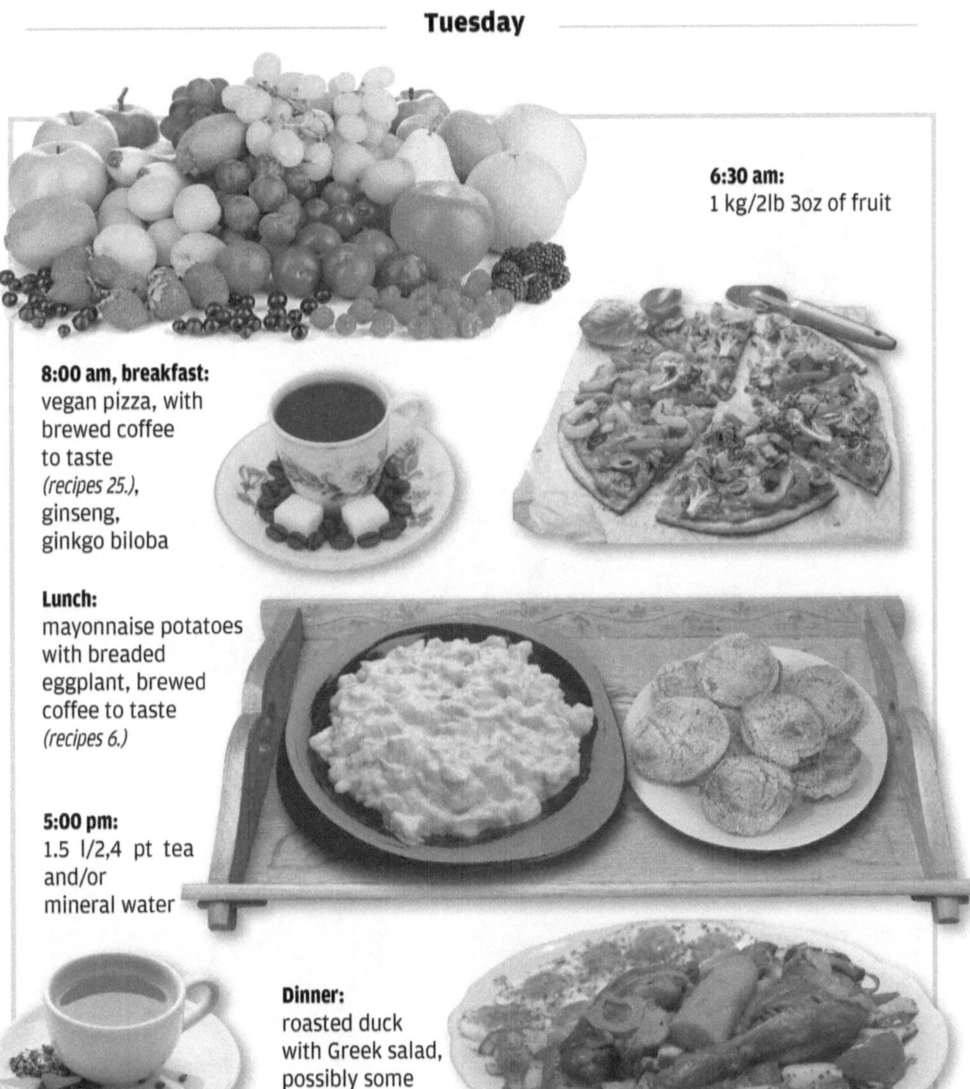

6:30 am:
1 kg/2lb 3oz of fruit

8:00 am, breakfast:
vegan pizza, with
brewed coffee
to taste
(recipes 25.),
ginseng,
ginkgo biloba

Lunch:
mayonnaise potatoes
with breaded
eggplant, brewed
coffee to taste
(recipes 6.)

5:00 pm:
1.5 l/2,4 pt tea
and/or
mineral water

Dinner:
roasted duck
with Greek salad,
possibly some
fried eggs
(recipes 11., 1.)

Blood Group A

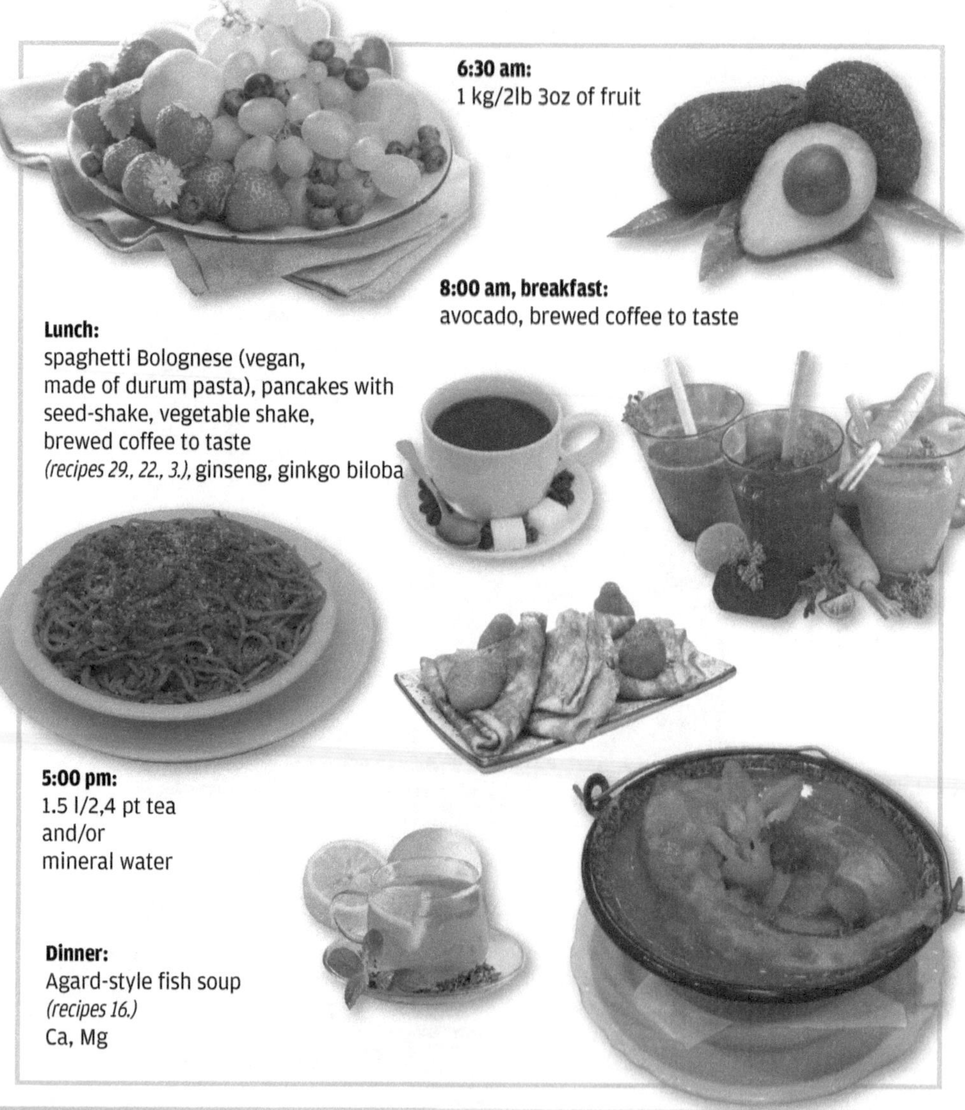

6:30 am:
1 kg/2lb 3oz of fruit

8:00 am, breakfast:
avocado, brewed coffee to taste

Lunch:
spaghetti Bolognese (vegan,
made of durum pasta), pancakes with
seed-shake, vegetable shake,
brewed coffee to taste
(recipes 29., 22., 3.), ginseng, ginkgo biloba

5:00 pm:
1.5 l/2,4 pt tea
and/or
mineral water

Dinner:
Agard-style fish soup
(recipes 16.)
Ca, Mg

Blood Group A

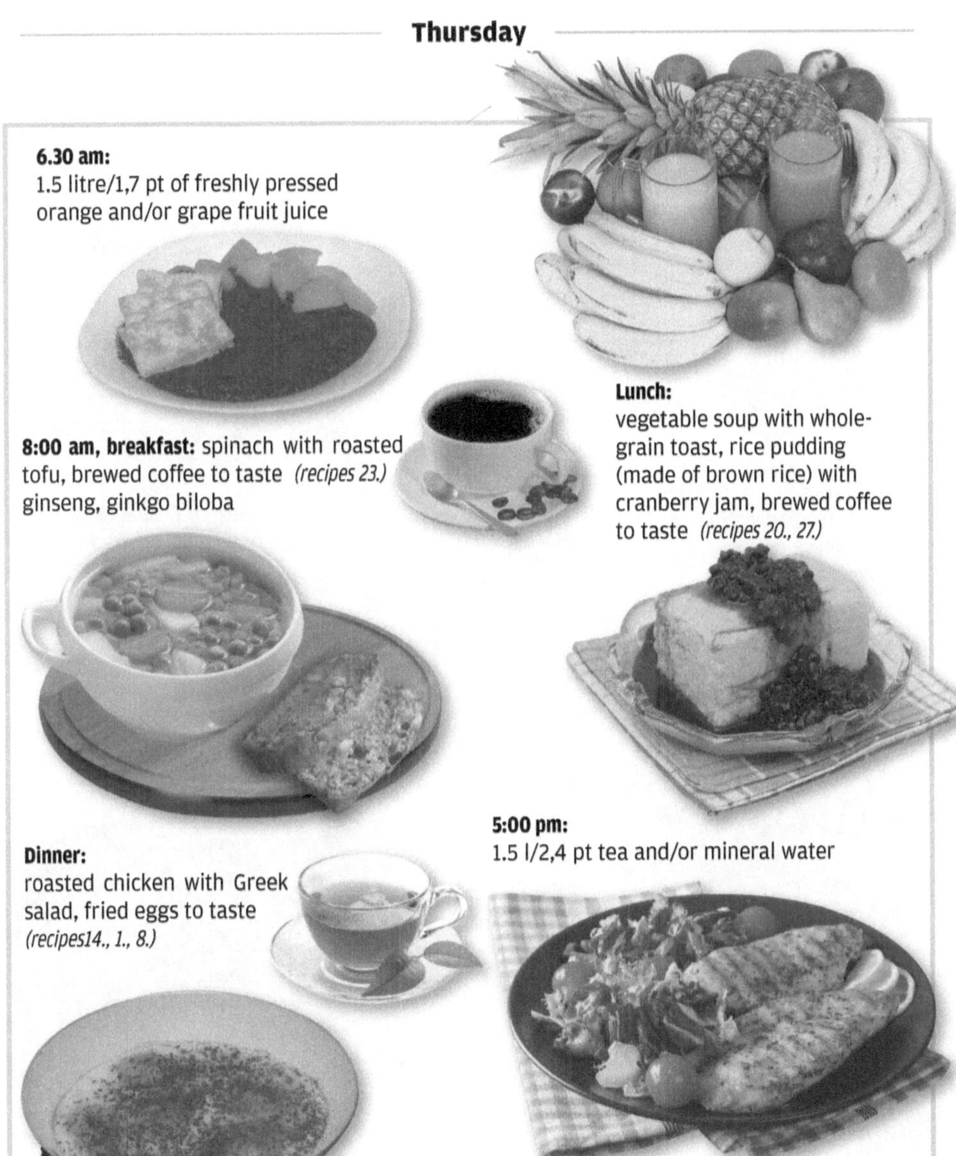

6.30 am:
1.5 litre/1,7 pt of freshly pressed orange and/or grape fruit juice

8:00 am, breakfast: spinach with roasted tofu, brewed coffee to taste *(recipes 23.)* ginseng, ginkgo biloba

Lunch:
vegetable soup with whole-grain toast, rice pudding (made of brown rice) with cranberry jam, brewed coffee to taste *(recipes 20., 27.)*

Dinner:
roasted chicken with Greek salad, fried eggs to taste *(recipes14., 1., 8.)*

5:00 pm:
1.5 l/2,4 pt tea and/or mineral water

Blood Group A

Friday

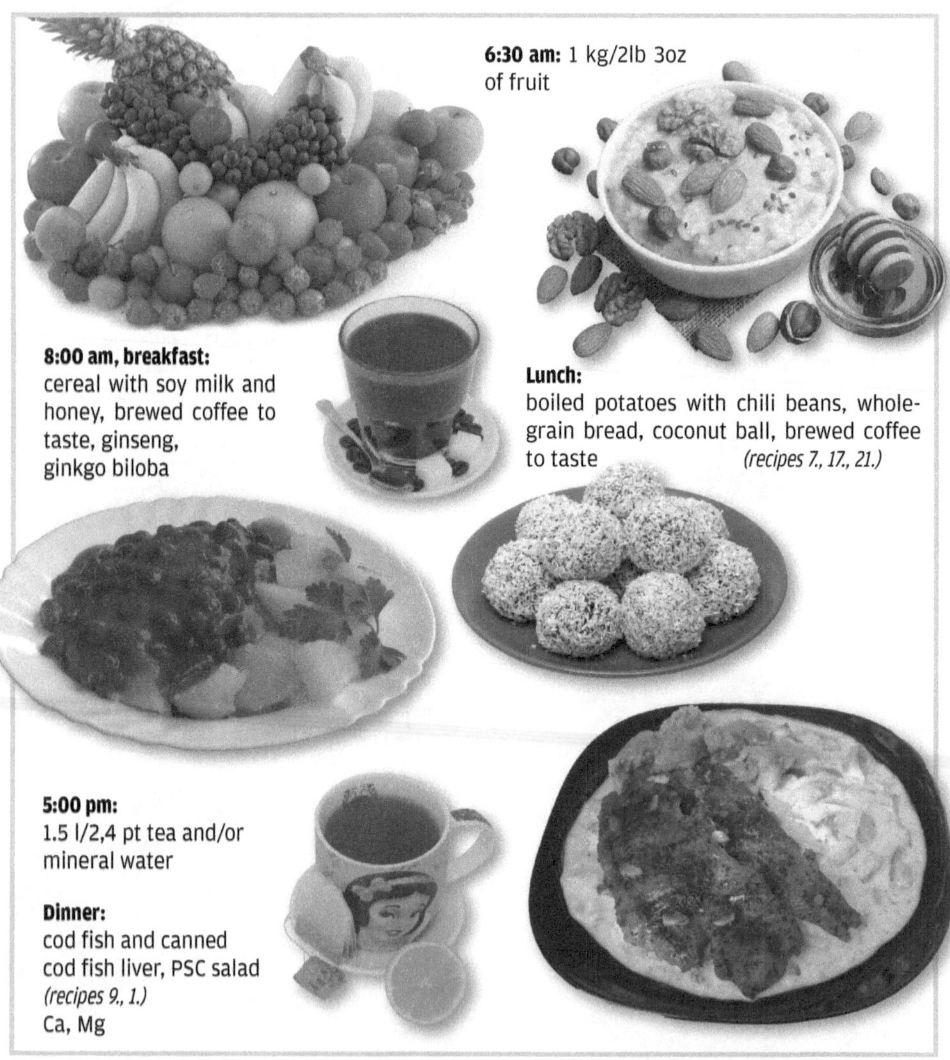

6:30 am: 1 kg/2lb 3oz of fruit

8:00 am, breakfast:
cereal with soy milk and honey, brewed coffee to taste, ginseng, ginkgo biloba

Lunch:
boiled potatoes with chili beans, whole-grain bread, coconut ball, brewed coffee to taste *(recipes 7., 17., 21.)*

5:00 pm:
1.5 l/2,4 pt tea and/or mineral water

Dinner:
cod fish and canned cod fish liver, PSC salad *(recipes 9., 1.)*
Ca, Mg

Blood Group A

Saturday

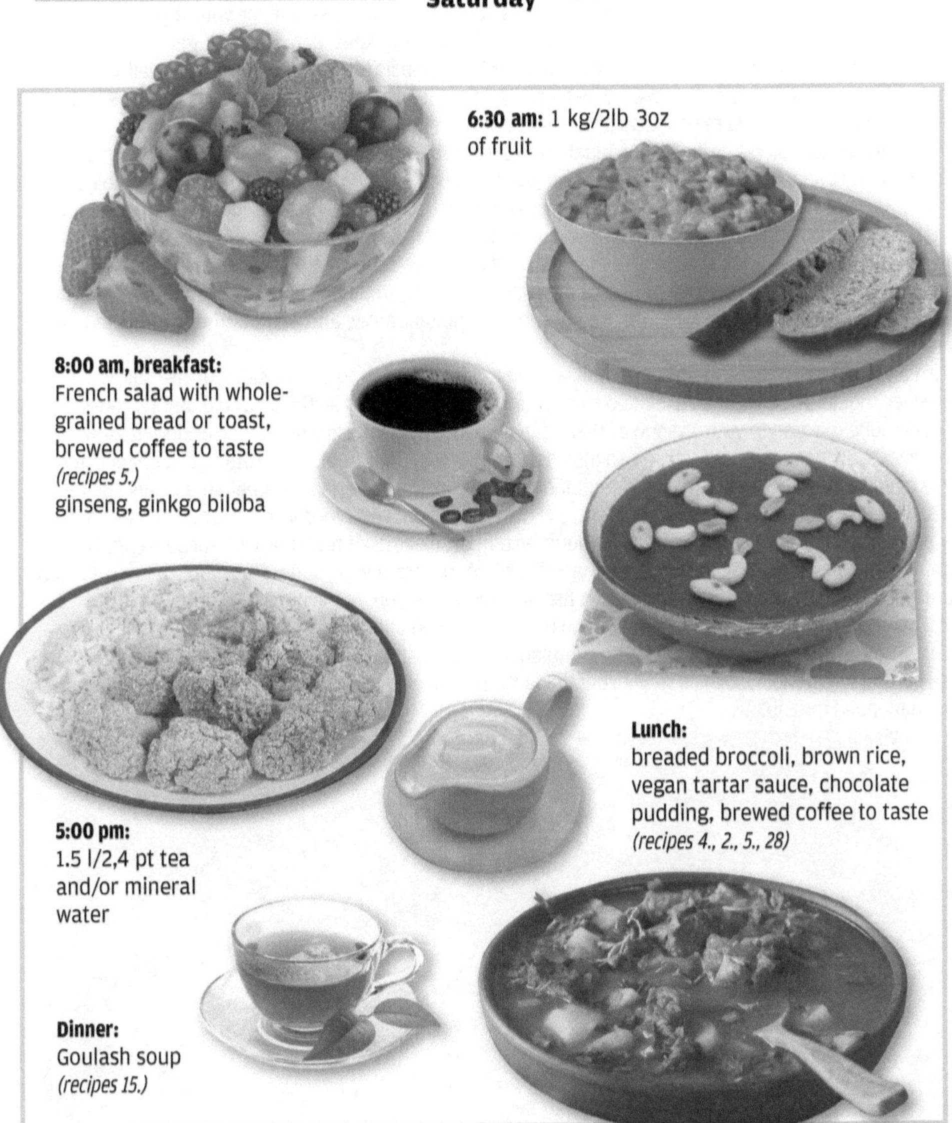

6:30 am: 1 kg/2lb 3oz of fruit

8:00 am, breakfast:
French salad with whole-grained bread or toast, brewed coffee to taste
(recipes 5.)
ginseng, ginkgo biloba

Lunch:
breaded broccoli, brown rice, vegan tartar sauce, chocolate pudding, brewed coffee to taste
(recipes 4., 2., 5., 28)

5:00 pm:
1.5 l/2,4 pt tea and/or mineral water

Dinner:
Goulash soup
(recipes 15.)

Blood Group B

People with type B blood carry the dominant genes of our livestock-breeding ancestors, who lived in the Caucasian Steppes, pasturing their herds, eating their meat and drinking their milk, while gathering wild plants. Due to their traveling lifestyle, they became the pioneers of global trading. If you have this blood type, activities that demand both strength and stamina are suitable for you such as rowing, cycling, or tennis. You have talents for business and languages. Citrus fruits are essential for your digestive system. As well as these, ripe and alkaline fruits are favorable: bananas, grapes, dates, and plums.

Contrary to other blood groups, blood group B and AB individuals tolerate dairy products well since they possess the enzymes required for their digestion in adulthood. Apart from that, blood group B individuals do well enough without dairy products as they are not essential for their metabolism.

There are certain blood group B individuals who are specifically milk-sensitive. Your lunch, similarly to blood group O, should consist of widely-grown grains such as brown rice, oats, rye, and vegetables. However, your ancestors probably often prepared it with milk back in their time, so for easier digestion, you had better avoid using milk for it. For dinner you should alternate fish with meat of herd animals such as sheep, goat, and cow, adding vegetables to meat dishes. Never consume milk with red meat, as they are completely indigestible together. Mammal meat abounds with iron, which induces a chemical reaction with the calcium found in milk if both are consumed simultaneously, and none of the benefits of either meat or milk can be utilized.

Fish and poultry are consumable with milk and eggs without any unpleasant side effects. Chicken meat however should be completely excluded from your diet, as it contains lectin in large quantity, causing an autoimmune reaction to you. As soon as this lectin goes into the bloodstream, B-type antibodies found on red blood cells perceive this lectin as an intruder, so they stick to it to block it. Afterward, phagocytes (a type of cell within the body capable of engulfing and absorbing bacteria and other small cells and particles) devour all these lectins together with your own red blood cells in order to accomplish their mission by perishing together. Therefore, your immune system destroys itself together with these lectins broken down from chicken meat, draining a vast amount of energy from your body. You should rather dine on turkey if you desire poultry. Consuming sea fish is essential for you, but avoid eating crab, shellfish, octopus, and calamari, as they are harmful due to toxins and some undesired and harmful proteins in them.

Cocoa, green and black teas are healthy stimulants for you instead of coffee which is not recommended. Use natural sweeteners, such as stevia containing 0 calories, or a daily maximum 1-2 tablespoon honey is recommended for you.

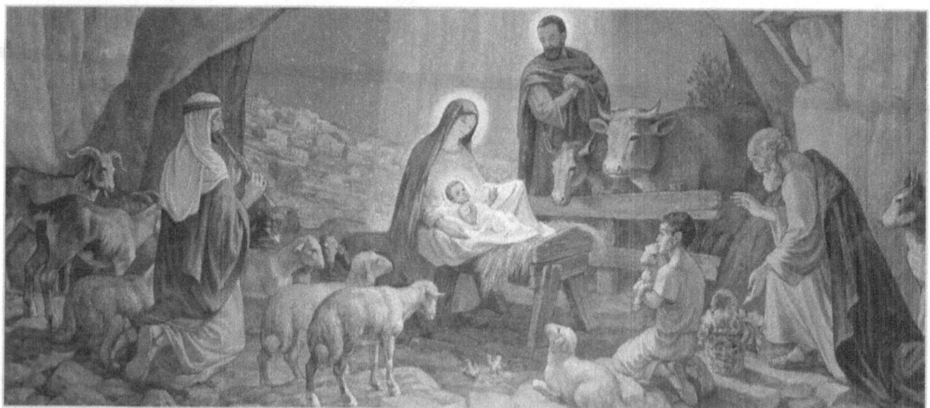

One Week Sample Diet for Blood Group B

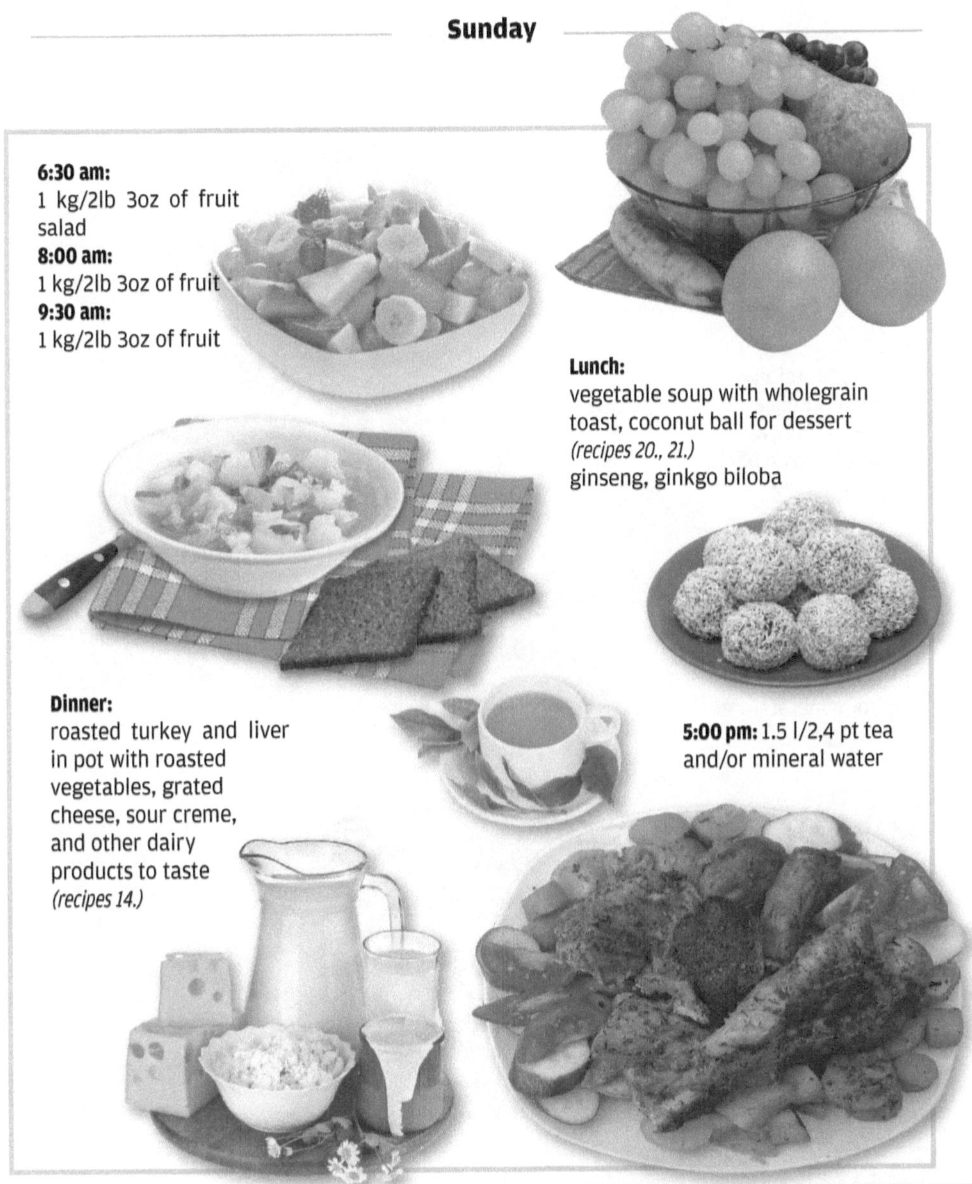

6:30 am:
1 kg/2lb 3oz of fruit salad
8:00 am:
1 kg/2lb 3oz of fruit
9:30 am:
1 kg/2lb 3oz of fruit

Lunch:
vegetable soup with wholegrain toast, coconut ball for dessert
(recipes 20., 21.)
ginseng, ginkgo biloba

Dinner:
roasted turkey and liver in pot with roasted vegetables, grated cheese, sour creme, and other dairy products to taste
(recipes 14.)

5:00 pm: 1.5 l/2,4 pt tea and/or mineral water

Blood Group B

6:30 am:
2 bananas, 2 apples
8: 00 am:
1 kg/2lb 3oz grape
9:30 am:
1 kg/2lb 3oz fruit

Lunch:
sweet-sour tofu with brown rice,
1 slice of wholegrain vegan pizza
(recipes 24., 25.)
ginseng, ginkgo biloba

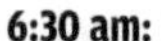

5:00 pm:
1.5 l/2,4 pt tea
and/or mineral water

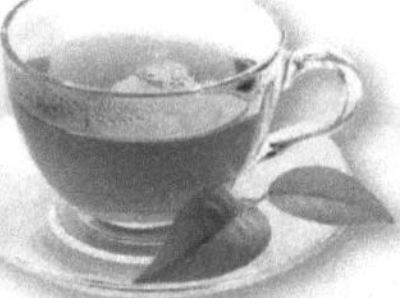

Dinner:
salmon, PBC salad,
possibly soft-boiled
eggs, dairy products
to taste
(recipes 14., 1.) Ca, Mg

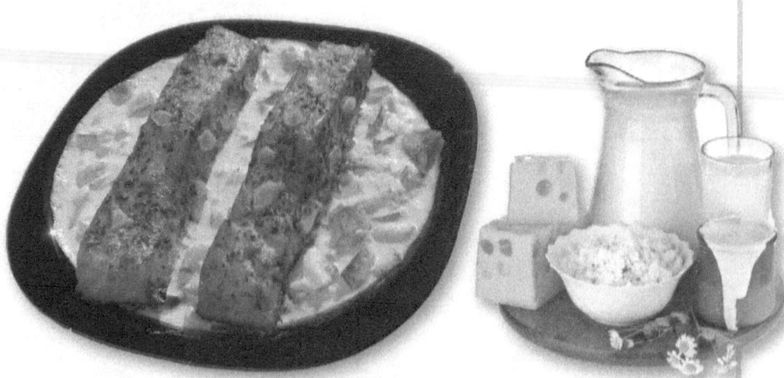

Blood Group B

Tuesday

6:30 am:
1 kg 1 kg/2lb 3oz fruit
8:00 am:
1 kg/2lb 3oz fruit
9:30 am:
1 kg/2lb 3oz fruit

Lunch:
mayonnaise
potatoes with
breaded broccoli
(recipes 6., 4.)
ginseng,
ginkgo biloba

5:00 pm:
1.5 l/2,4 pt tea
and/or mineral water

Dinner:
roasted lamb
with Greek salad
(recipes 14., 1.)

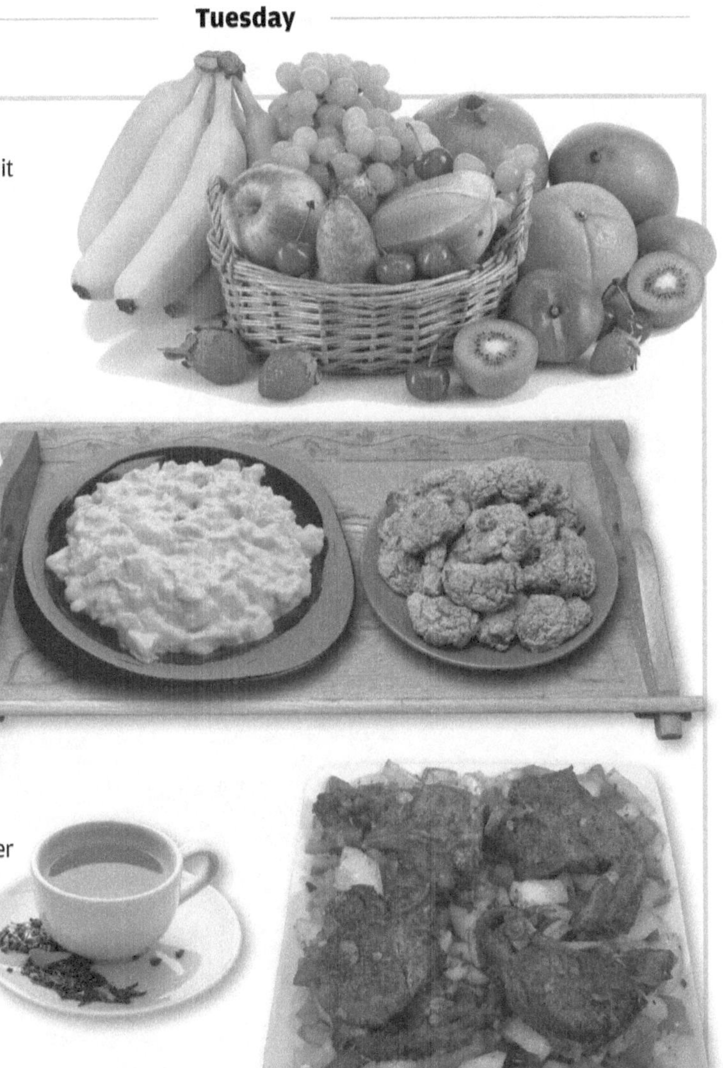

Blood Group B

Wendesday

6:30 am:
1 kg 1 kg/2lb 3oz fruit
8:00 am:
1 kg/2lb 3oz fruit
9:30 am:
1 kg/2lb 3oz fruit

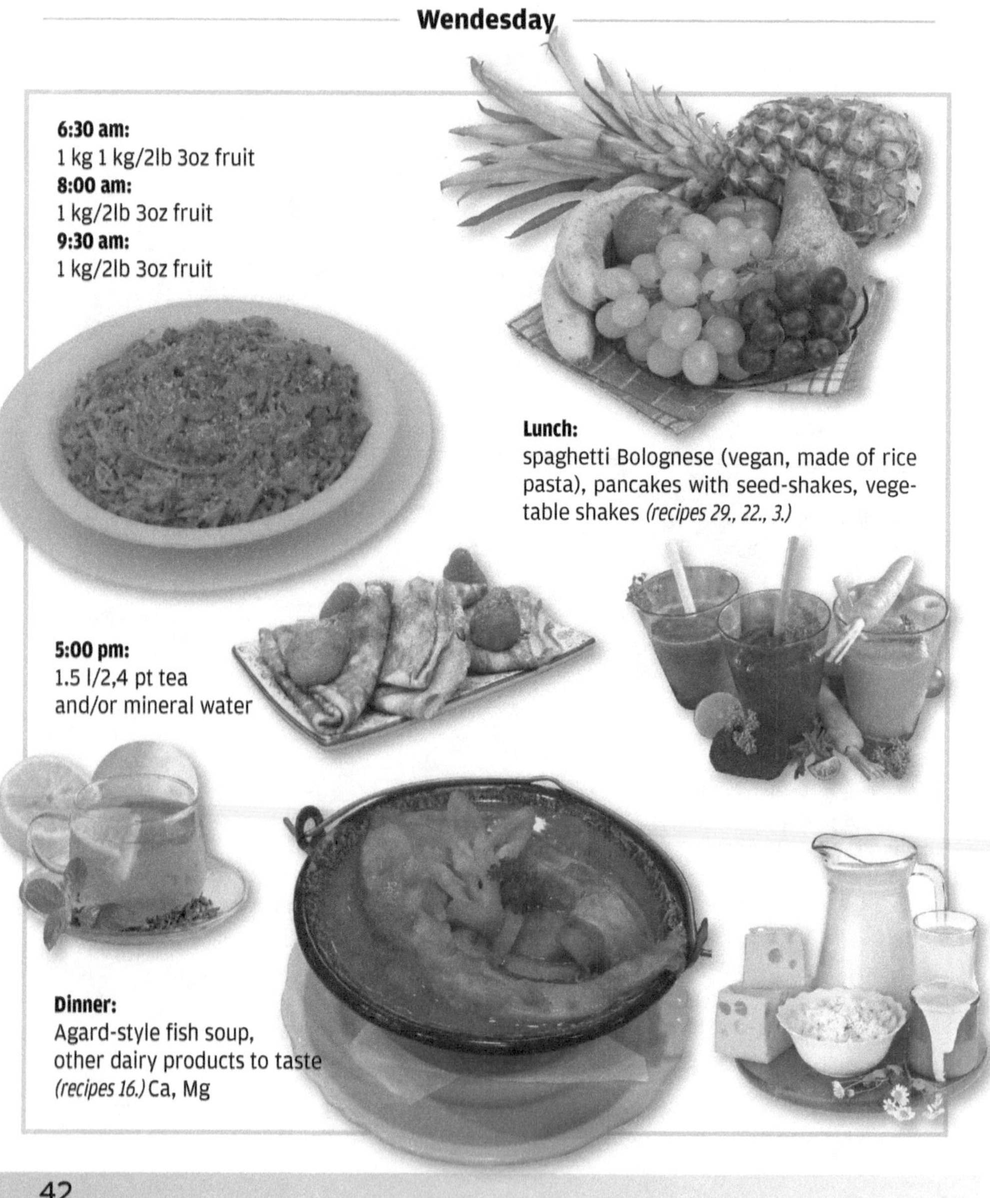

Lunch:
spaghetti Bolognese (vegan, made of rice pasta), pancakes with seed-shakes, vegetable shakes *(recipes 29., 22., 3.)*

5:00 pm:
1.5 l/2,4 pt tea
and/or mineral water

Dinner:
Agard-style fish soup,
other dairy products to taste
(recipes 16.) Ca, Mg

Blood Group B

Thursday

6.30 am:
1 l/1,7 pt fresh orange/grapefruit juice
8:00 am:
1 kg/2lb 3oz fruit
9.30 am:
1 kg/2lb 3oz fruit

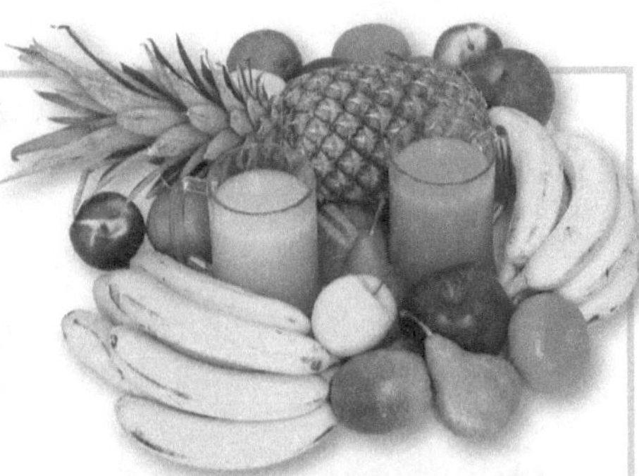

Lunch:
vegetable soup with wholegrain rye toast, rice pudding (made from brown rice) with cranberry jam, ginseng, ginko biloba *(recipes 20., 27.)*

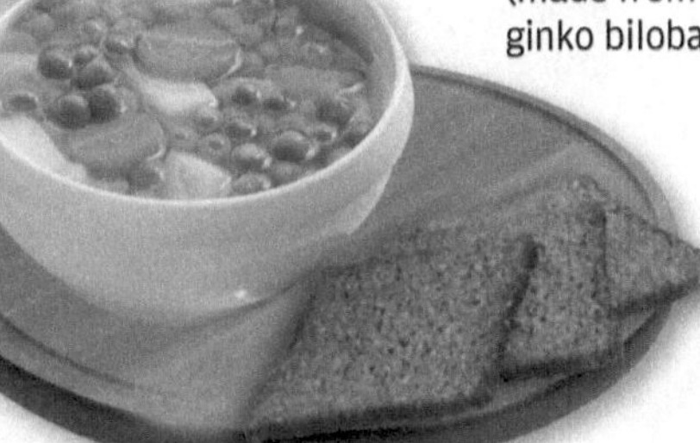

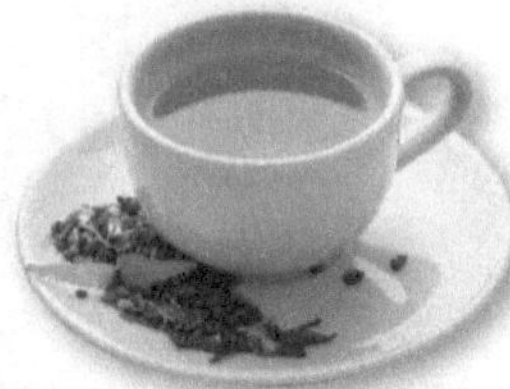

5:00 pm:
1.5 l/2,4 pt tea
and/or mineral water

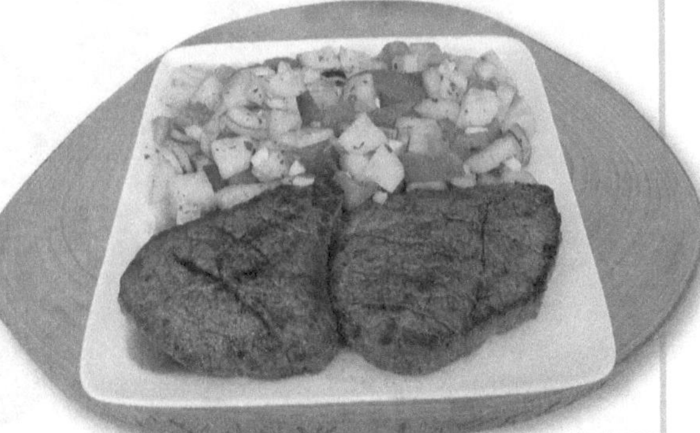

Dinner:
beef steak with Greek salad
(recipes 12., 1.)

Blood Group B

6.30 am:
1 kg/2lb 3oz fruit
8:00 am:
1 kg/2lb 3oz fruit
9.30 am:
1 kg/2lb 3oz fruit

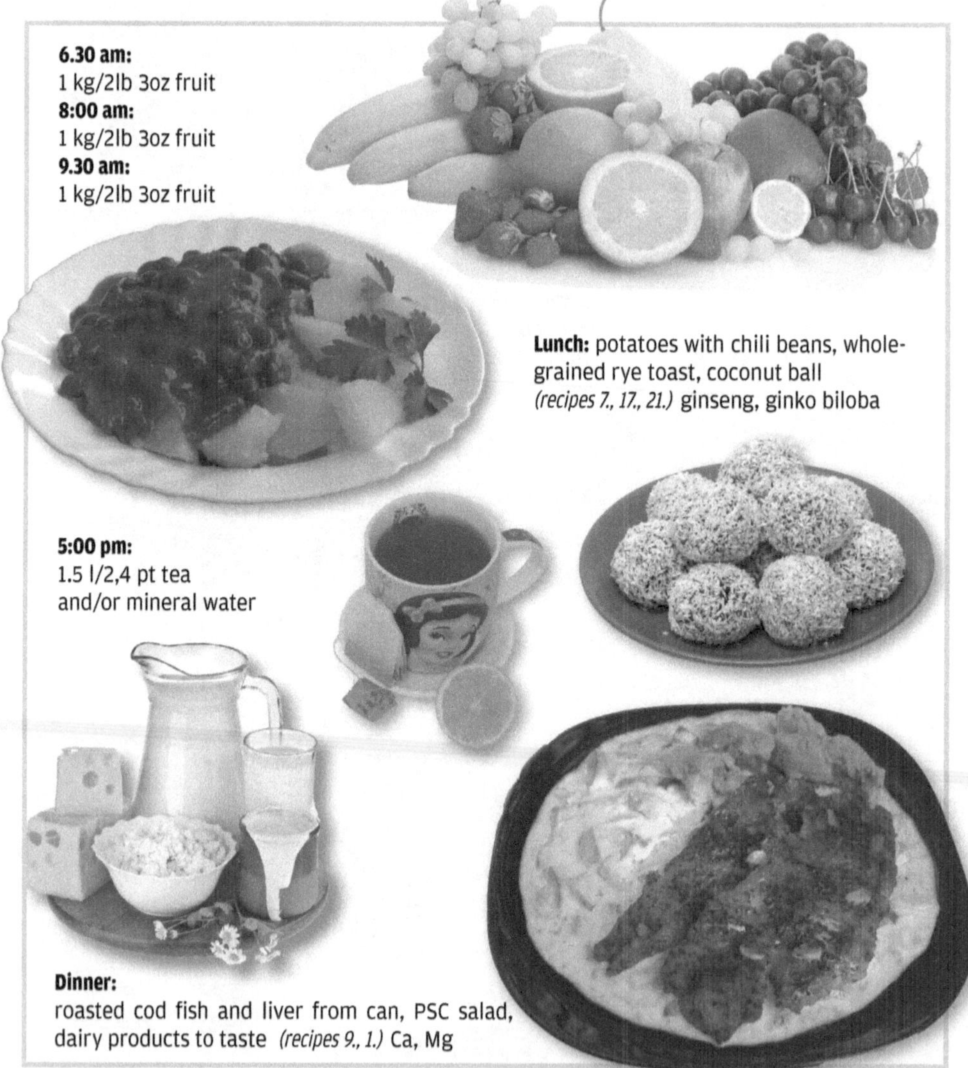

Lunch: potatoes with chili beans, whole-grained rye toast, coconut ball
(recipes 7., 17., 21.) ginseng, ginko biloba

5:00 pm:
1.5 l/2,4 pt tea
and/or mineral water

Dinner:
roasted cod fish and liver from can, PSC salad, dairy products to taste *(recipes 9., 1.)* Ca, Mg

Blood Group B

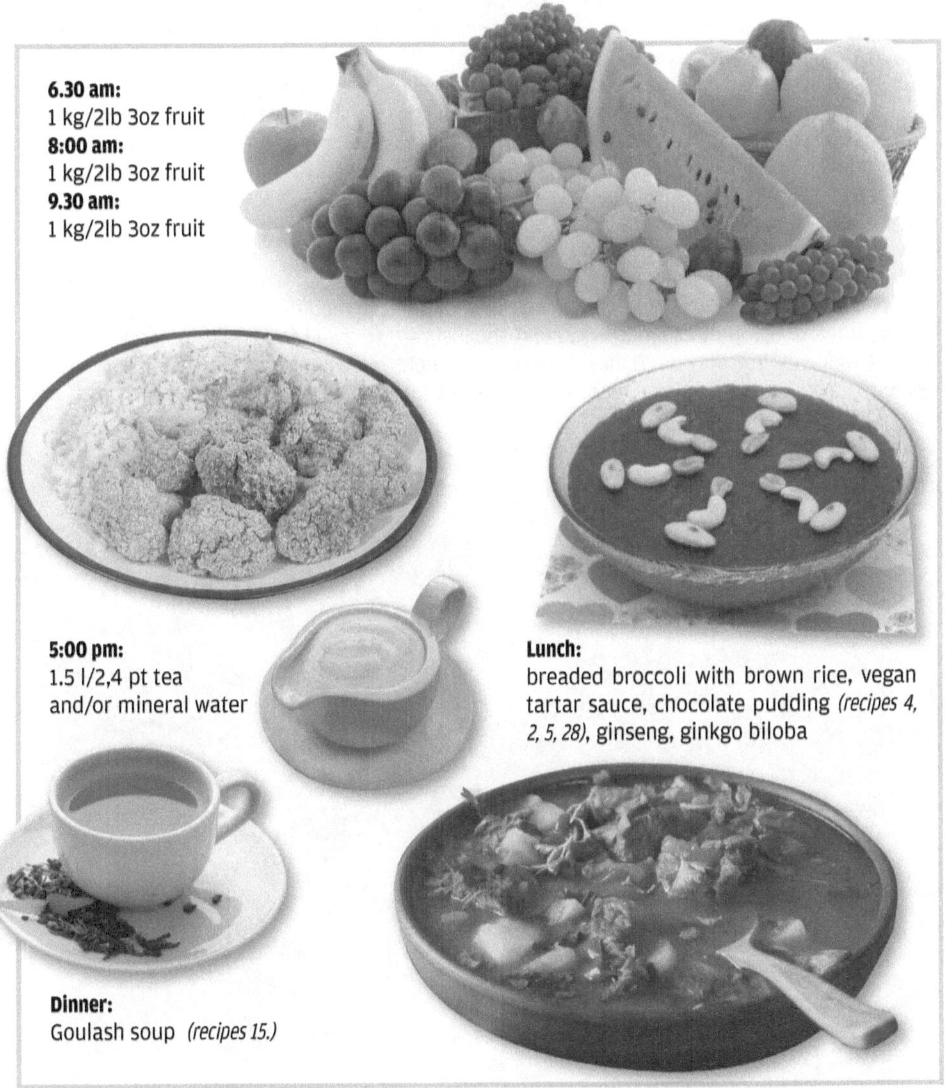

6.30 am:
1 kg/2lb 3oz fruit
8:00 am:
1 kg/2lb 3oz fruit
9.30 am:
1 kg/2lb 3oz fruit

Lunch:
breaded broccoli with brown rice, vegan tartar sauce, chocolate pudding *(recipes 4, 2, 5, 28)*, ginseng, ginkgo biloba

5:00 pm:
1.5 l/2,4 pt tea
and/or mineral water

Dinner:
Goulash soup *(recipes 15.)*

Blood Group AB:

People with type AB blood carry the dominant genes (or codominant in this case) of both our plant-cultivating and our livestock-breeding ancestors. You are a social person with great communication skills. You have the abilities of both blood group A and B individuals. However, all of their food intolerances are applicable to you. Hence for example, you should avoid consuming tomato and chicken.

You are fortunate since out of the four blood groups, your body is the most prepared for the abundance of foods that are available to us nowadays, which can cause diseases and obesity to people with other types of blood. Your red blood cells carry antibodies of both type A and B; therefore you are the most resistant to infectious diseases.

Your digestive system is prepared to handle any types of foods, so you can consume and easily digest all kinds of red meat, poultry, fish, eggs, leguminous plants, fruits, vegetables, grains, nuts, oily seeds and dairy products. Timing and pairing of foods is the only task for you, in order to avoid toxin production by heavy digestion. There are plenty of healthy protein sources for you, such as fish, beef, lamb, goat, or turkey; leguminous plants such as beans, soy, lentils and peas; and dairy products. Consume offal moderately. Your body - though requiring none - also tolerates animal fat and vegetable oil well.

Cocoa, tea, and traditional brewed coffee are all useful stimulants for you. Since you are subject to cancer, the intake of high-cholesterol foods should be much moderated. Avoid consuming pork, chicken, tomato, octopus, calamari, crab and shellfish, try to avoid foods with preservatives and artificial additives. You may use honey, natural sweeteners and even sugar to sweeten your dishes. Stevia is the best amongst them, as it is natural and contains 0 calories. Eat organic foods if possible.

Please read the chapters for blood groups A and B, since both are applicable to you.

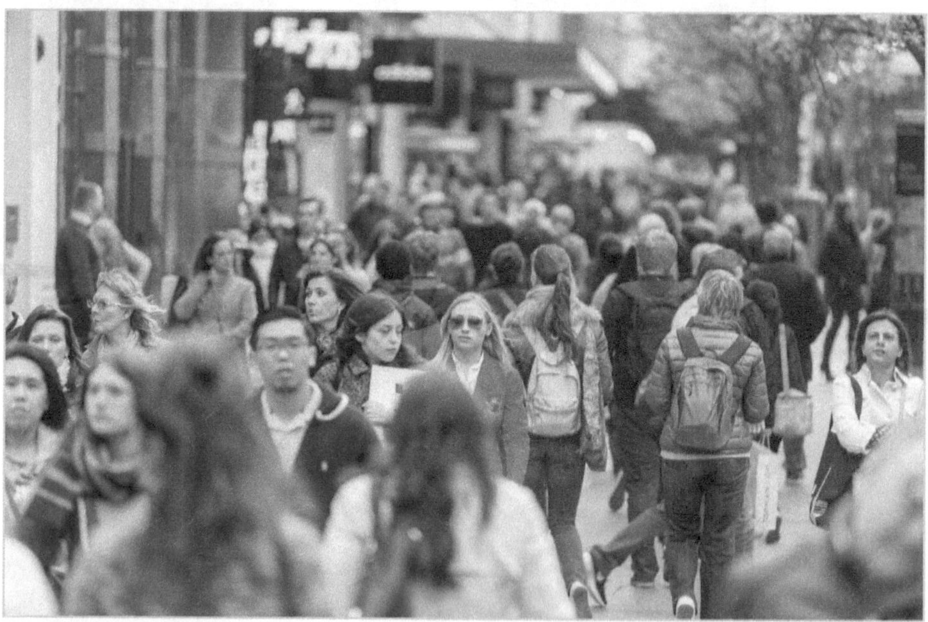

One Week Sample Diet for Blood Group AB

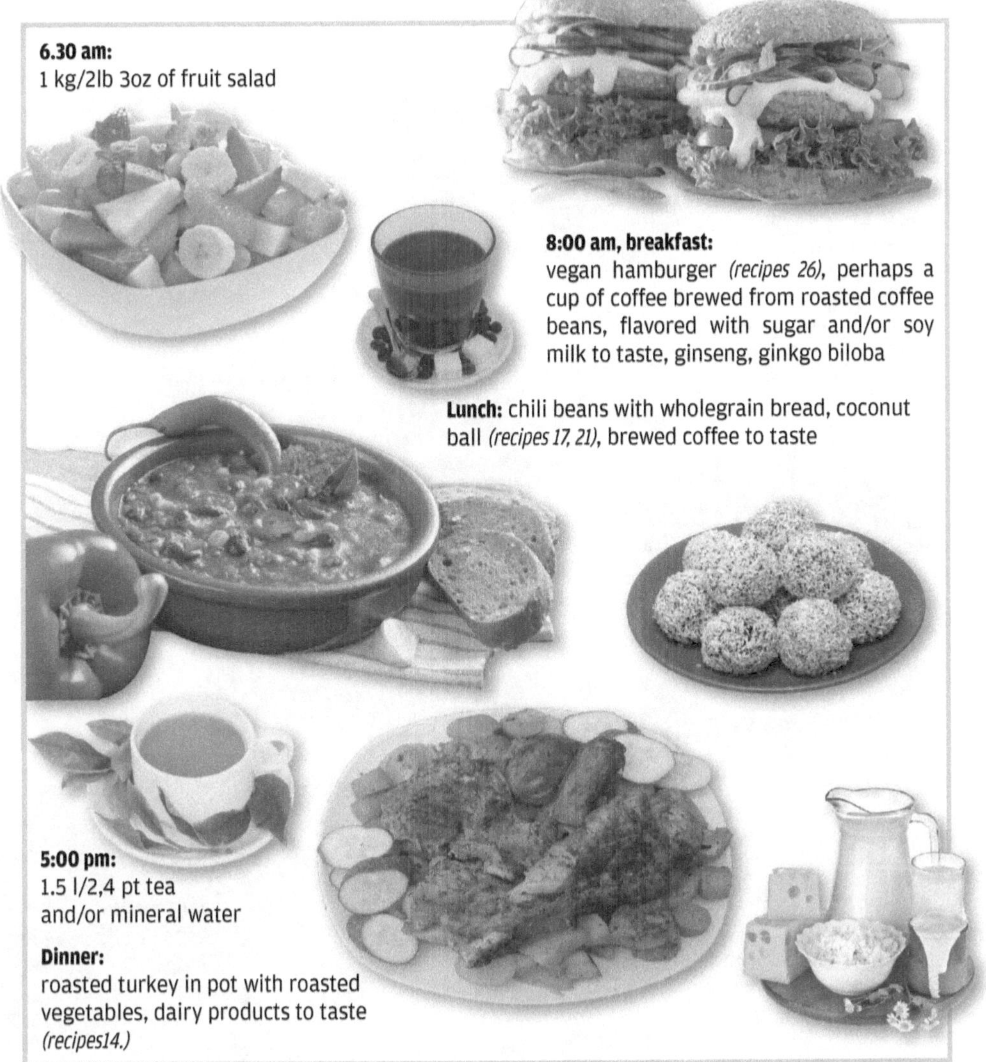

6.30 am:
1 kg/2lb 3oz of fruit salad

8:00 am, breakfast:
vegan hamburger *(recipes 26)*, perhaps a cup of coffee brewed from roasted coffee beans, flavored with sugar and/or soy milk to taste, ginseng, ginkgo biloba

Lunch: chili beans with wholegrain bread, coconut ball *(recipes 17, 21)*, brewed coffee to taste

5:00 pm:
1.5 l/2,4 pt tea
and/or mineral water

Dinner:
roasted turkey in pot with roasted vegetables, dairy products to taste
(recipes14.)

Blood Group AB

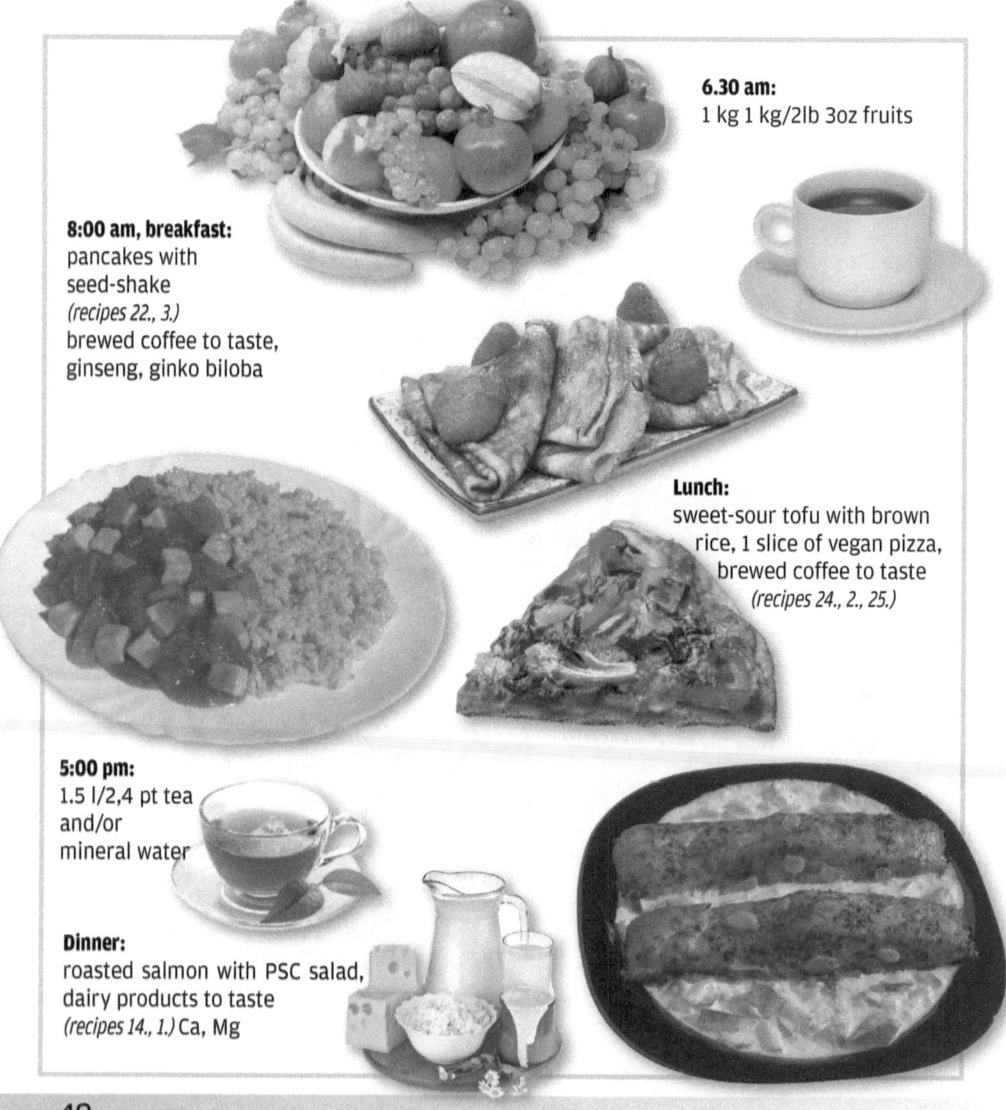

6.30 am:
1 kg 1 kg/2lb 3oz fruits

8:00 am, breakfast:
pancakes with
seed-shake
(recipes 22., 3.)
brewed coffee to taste,
ginseng, ginko biloba

Lunch:
sweet-sour tofu with brown
rice, 1 slice of vegan pizza,
brewed coffee to taste
(recipes 24., 2., 25.)

5:00 pm:
1.5 l/2,4 pt tea
and/or
mineral water

Dinner:
roasted salmon with PSC salad,
dairy products to taste
(recipes 14., 1.) Ca, Mg

Blood Group AB

Tuesday

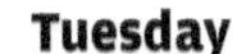

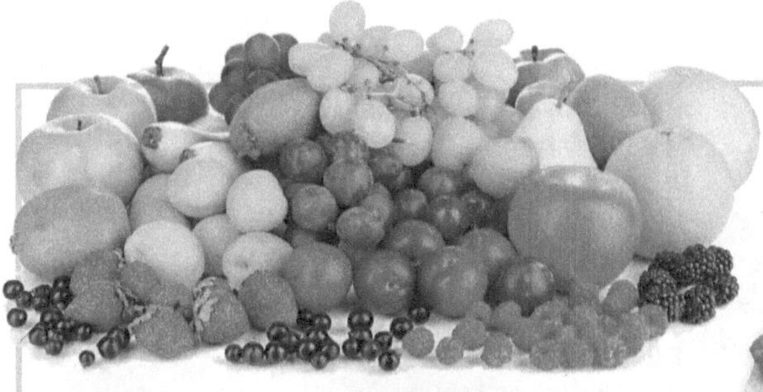

6.30 am:
1 kg 1 kg/2lb 3oz fruits

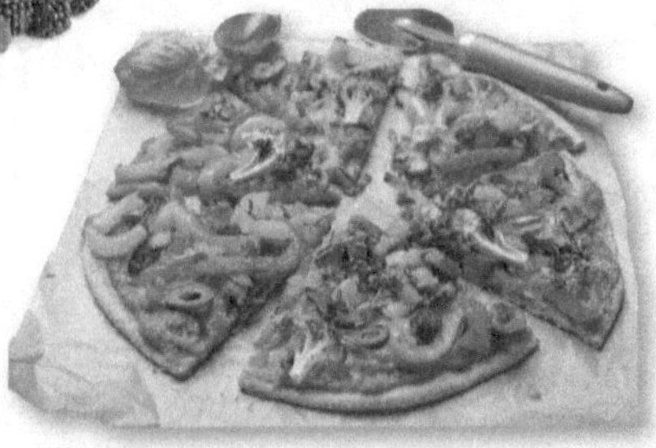

8:00 am, breakfast:
vegan pizza
(recipes 25..),
brewed coffee
to taste,
ginseng,
ginko biloba

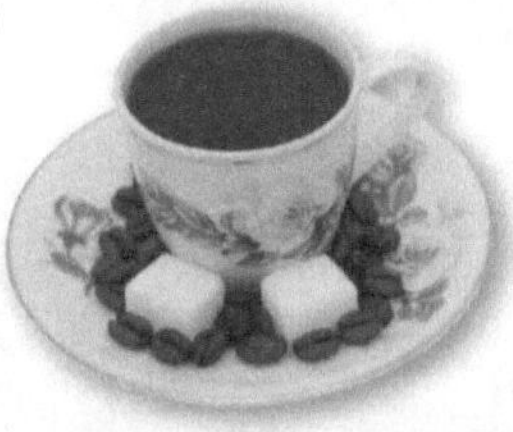

Lunch:
mayonnaise potatoes
with breaded
eggplant
(recipes 6., 4.),
brewed coffee
to taste

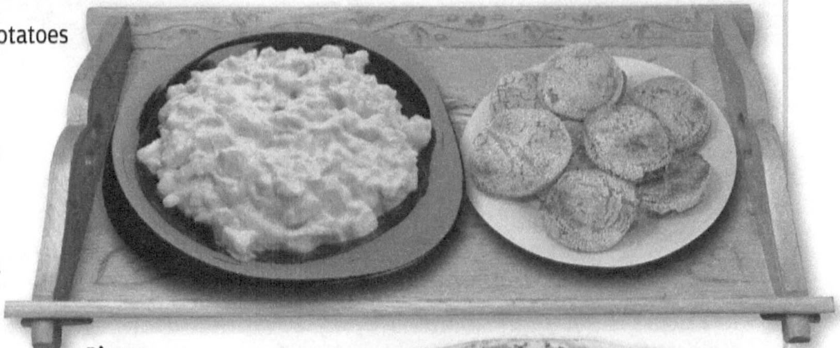

5:00 pm:
1.5 l/2,4 pt tea
and/or
mineral water

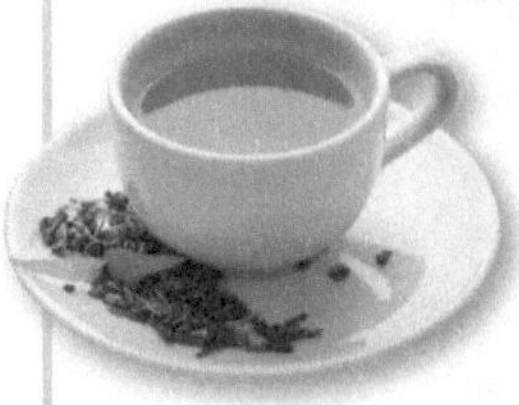

Dinner:
duck with
Greek salad,
possibly some fried
eggs, dairy
products to taste
(recipes 11., 1.)

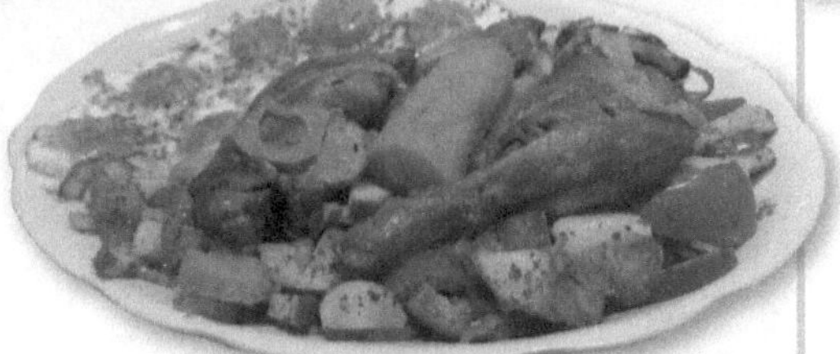

Blood Group AB

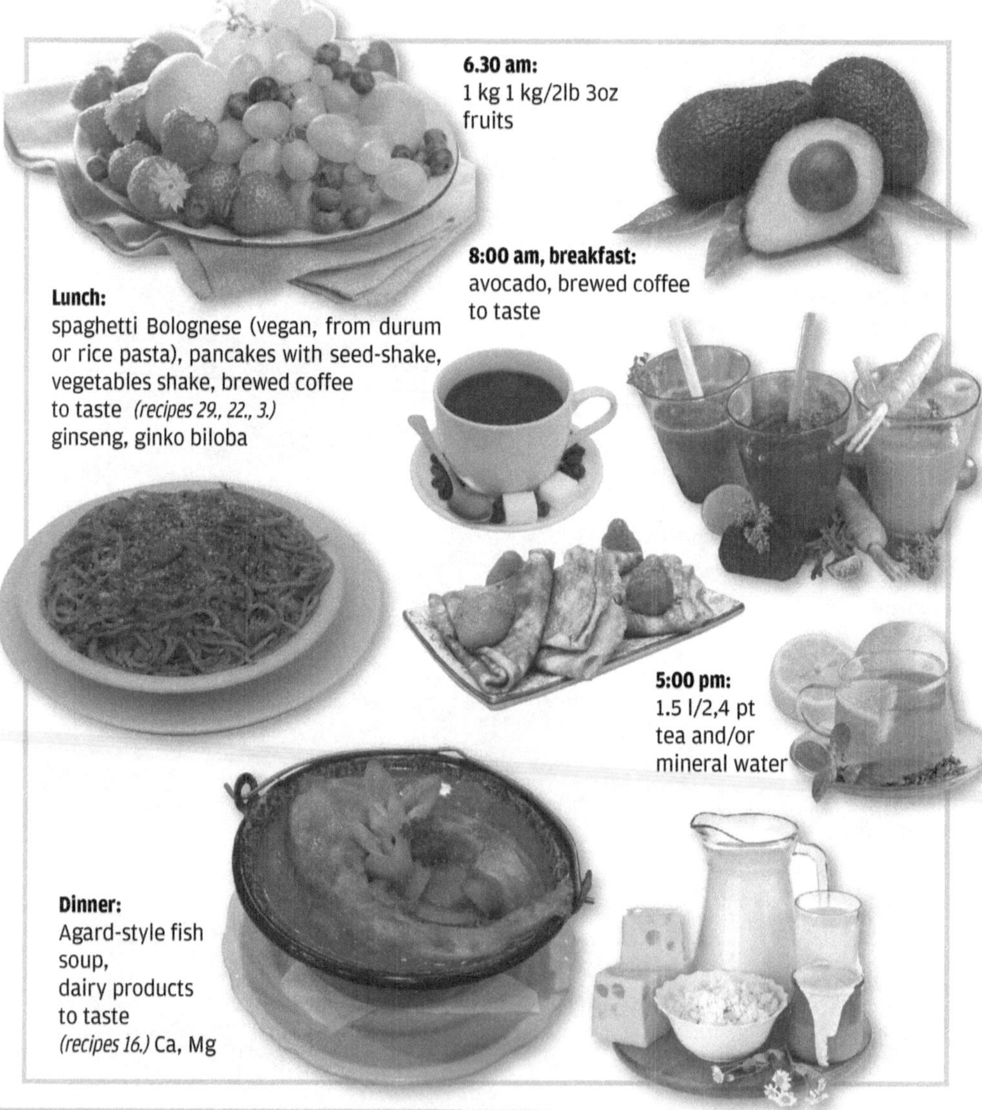

6.30 am:
1 kg 1 kg/2lb 3oz
fruits

8:00 am, breakfast:
avocado, brewed coffee
to taste

Lunch:
spaghetti Bolognese (vegan, from durum
or rice pasta), pancakes with seed-shake,
vegetables shake, brewed coffee
to taste *(recipes 29., 22., 3.)*
ginseng, ginko biloba

5:00 pm:
1.5 l/2,4 pt
tea and/or
mineral water

Dinner:
Agard-style fish
soup,
dairy products
to taste
(recipes 16.) Ca, Mg

Blood Group AB

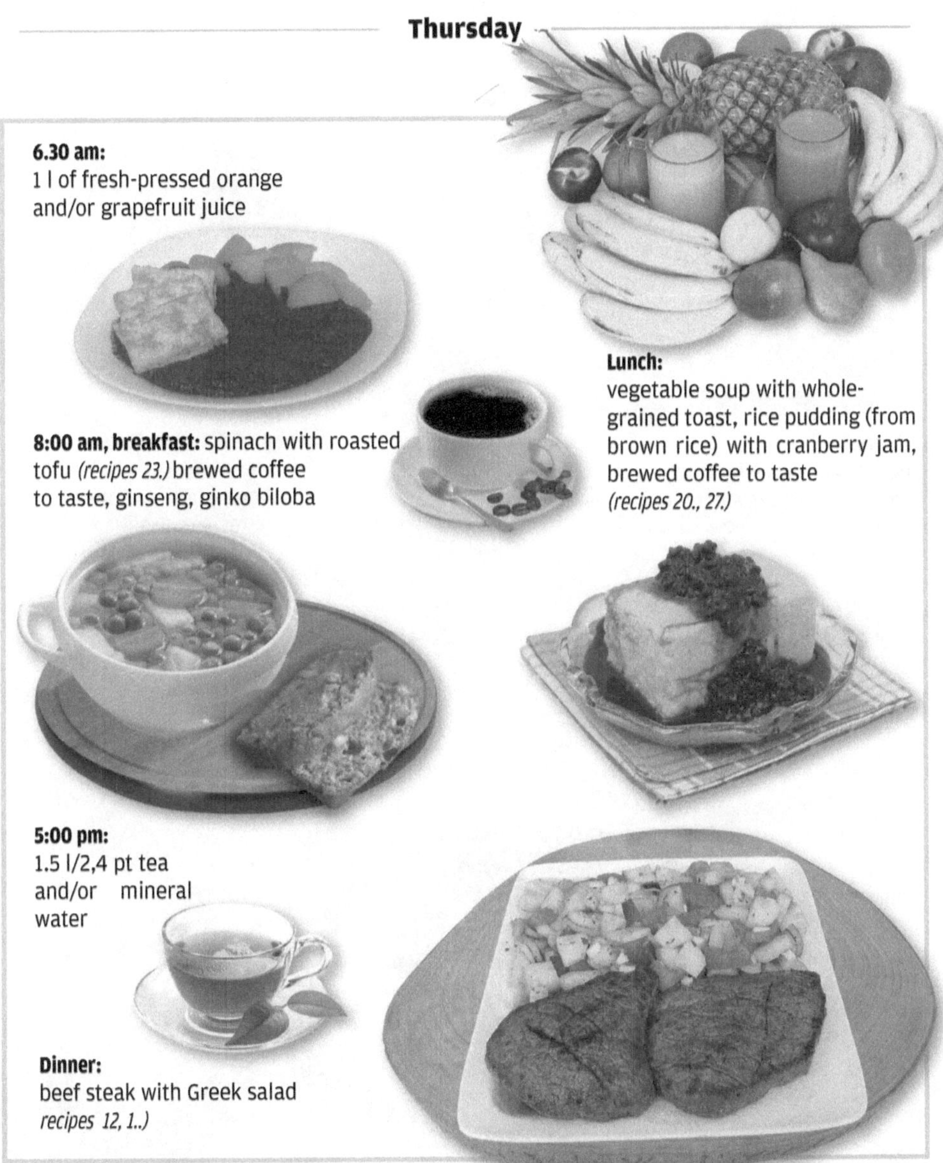

6.30 am:
1 l of fresh-pressed orange
and/or grapefruit juice

8:00 am, breakfast: spinach with roasted
tofu *(recipes 23.)* brewed coffee
to taste, ginseng, ginko biloba

Lunch:
vegetable soup with whole-
grained toast, rice pudding (from
brown rice) with cranberry jam,
brewed coffee to taste
(recipes 20., 27.)

5:00 pm:
1.5 l/2,4 pt tea
and/or   mineral
water

Dinner:
beef steak with Greek salad
recipes 12, 1..)

Blood Group AB

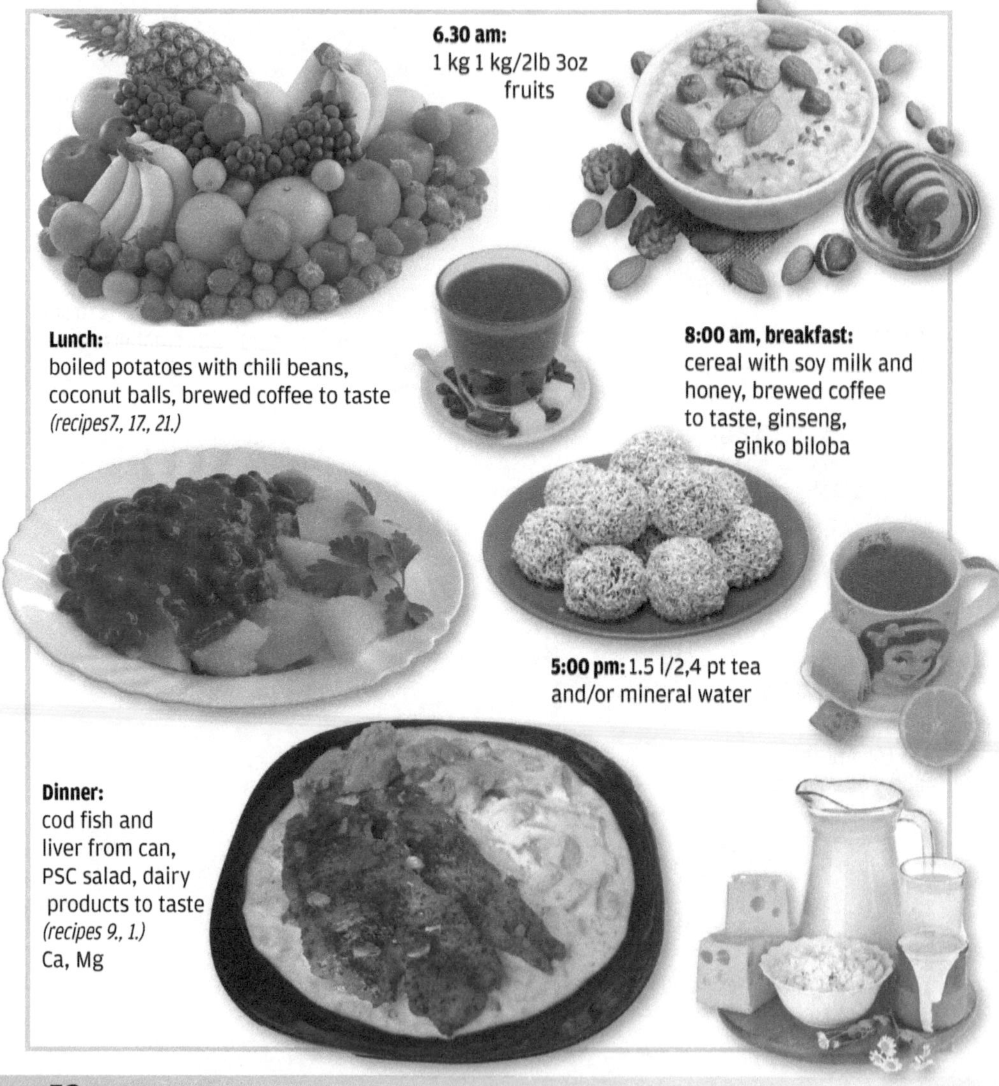

6.30 am:
1 kg 1 kg/2lb 3oz
fruits

8:00 am, breakfast:
cereal with soy milk and
honey, brewed coffee
to taste, ginseng,
ginko biloba

Lunch:
boiled potatoes with chili beans,
coconut balls, brewed coffee to taste
(recipes7., 17., 21.)

5:00 pm: 1.5 l/2,4 pt tea
and/or mineral water

Dinner:
cod fish and
liver from can,
PSC salad, dairy
 products to taste
(recipes 9., 1.)
Ca, Mg

Blood Group AB

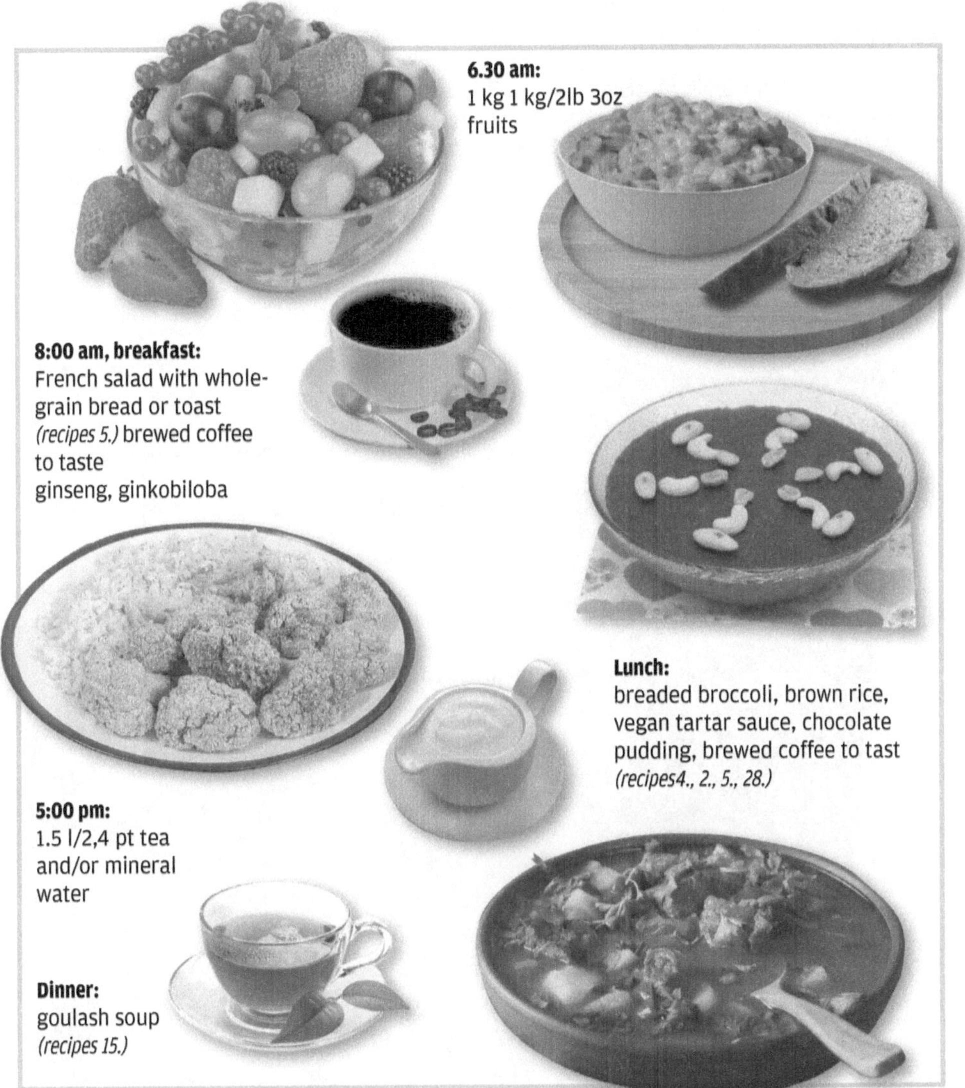

6.30 am:
1 kg 1 kg/2lb 3oz
fruits

8:00 am, breakfast:
French salad with whole-grain bread or toast
(recipes 5.) brewed coffee
to taste
ginseng, ginkobiloba

Lunch:
breaded broccoli, brown rice,
vegan tartar sauce, chocolate
pudding, brewed coffee to tast
(recipes4., 2., 5., 28.)

5:00 pm:
1.5 l/2,4 pt tea
and/or mineral
water

Dinner:
goulash soup
(recipes 15.)

Vegetable Oil and Animal Fat

Our body requires neither animal fat nor vegetable oil, although these have been a regular part of man's diet for many years.

These substances are especially fattening since they contain a large amount of empty calories while supplying no nutrients. Fish and even lean meat contain plenty of fat essential for the absorption of fat-soluble vitamins. When preparing your dishes, use as little fat as possible. Frying your meal in a thick ceramic pan is recommended since only a minimal amount of fat is required. Likewise, if fatty meat is fried sufficiently, the fat which melts out of it should be poured away and discarded at the end of cooking.

Sixty per cent of our brain consists of omega-3 and omega-6 polyunsaturated fatty acids, found mainly in deep-sea fishes. These fatty acids are essential for the operation of our brain and nervous system. Always fry fish in its own fat if possible or use fat from a fatty fish like salmon, using a ceramic pan. You can fry other less fatty fish using this melted fat afterwards. Using cod liver oil or butter is also possible, however, roasting fish in the oven is the simplest way to prepare it. Fish fat is well-tolerated by all blood groups. Fish fat is necessary but consume only as much as contained in the prepared fish, no more.

People with blood types O and B are much more tolerant of animal fat than of vegetable oil, so the latter often causes obesity and cardiovascular diseases for them. Conversely, the opposite is true of people with type A blood. Their body is more tolerant of vegetable oil than animal fat, which can cause diseases and weight gain.

Although blood group A individuals do not require vegetable oil, they do need essential amino acids, enzymes, minerals and vitamins found in oily seeds, the vegetable oil content of which is well-tolerated by them. Except in the case of olive oil, cooking with vegetable oil is dangerous and harmful to our health since heating transforms vegetable oil into trans-fats. This

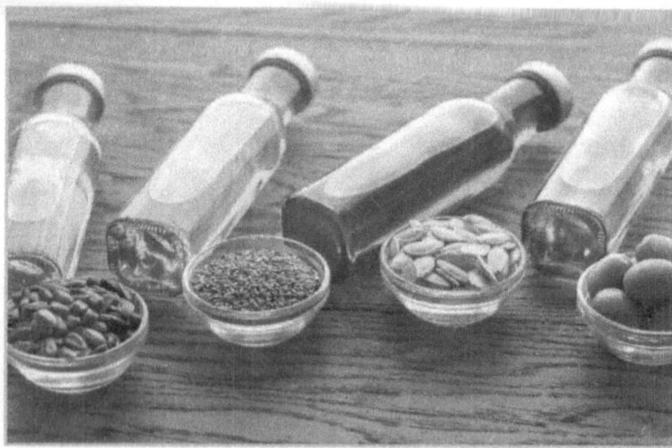

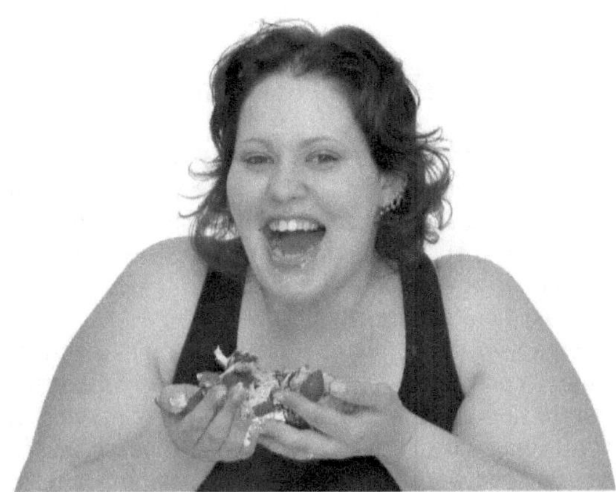

s, forming an anchor-like shape. These anchors hook onto the surface of our veins, disturbing healthy circulation by obstructing blood flow, thereby causing cardiovascular diseases.

Hot-pressed oil, besides trans-fat, contains traces of the petroleum oil used for the lubrication of hot-press machines. By using hot-press machines, 40-50% more oil is produced than by cold-pressing. This is the reason why hot-pressed oils are cheaper. Although considering only small amounts, sensitive people may face severe health problems using hot-pressed oil, since petroleum oil is amongst the most environmentally pollutant substances on Earth.

Don't save money on more expensive, cold-pressed oil! It is even better if we consume just oily seeds. Margarine and most chocolates are made from cheaper vegetable oils, which are prepared by a process called hydrogenation that transforms vegetable oils to solid trans-fat, contributing to cardiovascular diseases for people especially with type O and B blood. Hot-pressed oil is inherently full of trans-fat.

For this reason, it is better to fry fish or meat in its own fat, or we may prepare fish or poultry dishes using butter. Virgin olive oil is likewise an option for blood group A and AB individuals. Reduce fat and oil consumption as much as possible! If a dish is prepared in fat, leave it on a paper towel which will absorb unnecessary fat used for frying. Roasting on barbecues helps to remove fat from fatty food. Never use a microwave oven, it destroys most of the nutriments in the food.

Nevertheless, if you are not subject to obesity, using fat that is well-tolerated by your blood group will not harm you severely, so you do not need to worry too much about removing it from your dish. It is worth noting that animal fat and vegetable oil are easily digestible with both animal proteins and complex carbohydrates.

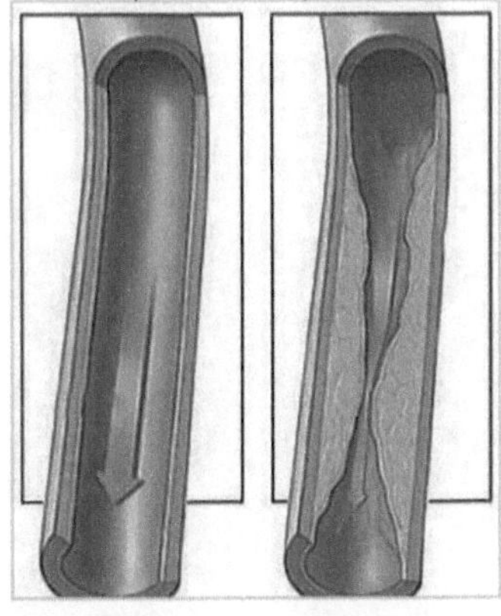

Healthly vein   Clogged vein

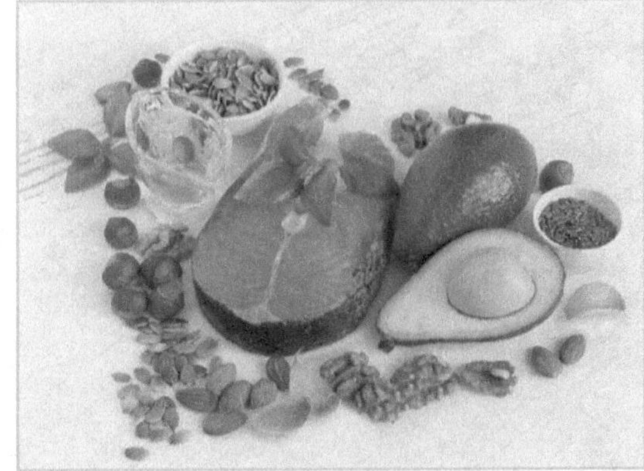

Healthy foods with high oil and fat content (they are also fattening)

The Acid-Base Balance of Our Body – Key to Losing Weight Permanently

You have probably heard that some substances such as foodstuffs, liquids, or our own body have a certain value known as the pH level. This shows the acidity of an aqueous solution. The scale goes from 0 to 14, where 0 indicates the most acidic substance, 14 the most alkaline, and 7 the neutral substances. Fewer free electrons in a substance means it is more acidic, more free electrons means it is more alkaline. So the more alkaline a substance is, the more electric energy and charge it has. Batteries operate based on this principle as well.

The human body is a highly complex bio-organism. Our brain operates with a micro-current, and through our nervous system, we are able to contract and move our muscles with assistance of this micro-current. In our sensory and motor nerves, as well as in our vegetative nervous system, the micro-current carries signals, controlling our digestive system, heartbeat, breathing and movement. Thus, the electric charge of our body, or its pH value, indicates the amount of energy we actually possess, not the quantity of consumed calories.

So, in order to energize ourselves, we need to alkalize our body. If we are sufficiently alkalized, we are full of energy, and our body can get rid of acidic toxins stored in fatty tissues and neutralize harmful acidic compounds. Furthermore, our body can regenerate itself faster and becomes more active with increased physical endurance and strength. Also, our resistance against diseases significantly improves, prolonging the lifetime of our cells together with our own life.

On the other hand, if our body is acidic, toxins (acids) cannot be neutralized but will be stored in fatty tissues instead, attempting to maintain the acid-base balance of the body.

Now we will examine what acidifies our body and drains us of life-force, and what alkalizes it and gives us strength to live.

The most significant acidifying factor is bad digestion, for example in the case of the simultaneous consumption of animal protein together with complex carbohydrates. The pH value of a consumed meal is likewise an important factor, as well as the biochemical reactions induced by various foods depending on your blood type. This is important since foods unsuitable for your blood type, even if they are alkaline, usually have an acidifying effect on you due to certain

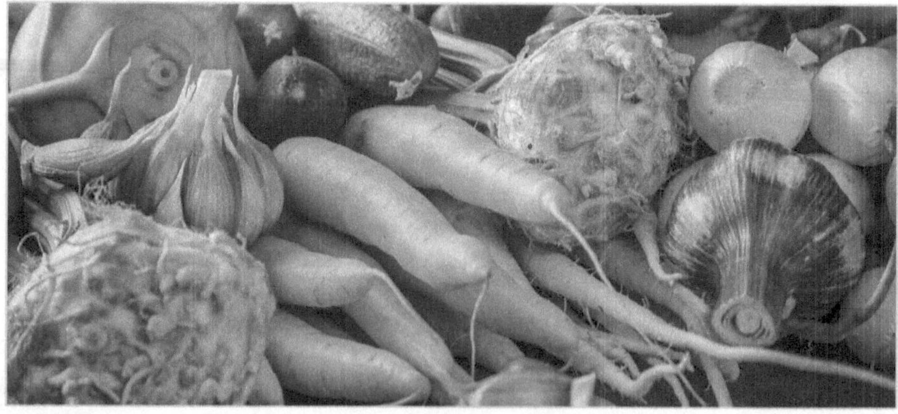

complex biochemical processes. This highlights the importance of consuming those foods that are compatible with your type of blood. Also, eat as wide a range of vegetables as possible!

Most vegetables, unlike other foodstuffs, are strongly alkaline. If you wish to alkalize yourself, drink a vegetable smoothie after your meal or simply eat more vegetables. Riper and sweeter fruits with higher sugar content such as banana, grape, and plum are slightly alkaline as well. If you desire to lose weight, the best way is to alkalize your body in order to use the energy surplus for physical exercise, burning unnecessary calories. As a result, alkalization prevents obesity. Pineapple, green tea and ginger consumption help slimming. Our kidneys can empty acids from the body through the urine, thus increased hydration further facilitates the alkalization.

Each animal protein such as meat, fish, eggs and dairy products are slightly acidic, but they are required by our body. Vegetables consumed with them are more alkaline, neutralizing the acidifying effect of the animal proteins.

You should try to avoid pork as it can contains worms and a high amount of uric acid, thus it is very acidifying. In the flesh and musculature of pigs lives a certain parasitic worm, called the pork tapeworm (taenia solium), which lives off the flesh of the animal, leaving its strongly acidic excrement behind. Hence, due to the feces of these worms, pork is high in toxins and uric acid.

The pig is genetically one of our closest relatives in the animal kingdom, thus pork consumption is slightly similar to the consumption of human flesh, and we are subject to infection by its tapeworms. Therefore, pork is not really suitable for humans.

Similarly, vinegar is an acid, having a strong acidifying effect on us. Thus, for preparing our salads, use freshly squeezed lemon juice instead. It is just as sour without being acidifying. Also, avoid sparkling drinks, as they contain carbon dioxide and other acids too. Amongst stimulants, green tea is neutral, while black tea and coffee are slightly acidic. Take care to remove teabags from your tea as advised on the packaging; otherwise the leaching tannin will acidify the tea strongly.

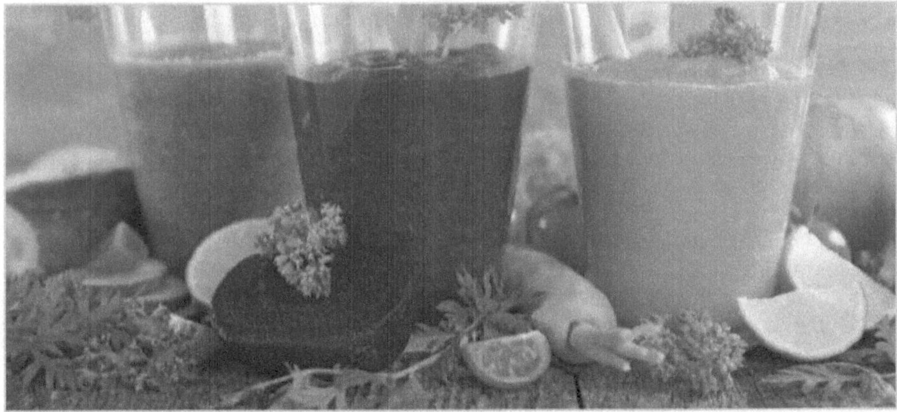

Introducing the Perfect Self Control System (PSC) into Your Diet

 Because healthy nutrition is based on very complex principles, please read this publication, Perfect Self Control, at least three times to learn all the main recommendations. Unfortunately, there are plenty of half-truths and misbeliefs around healthy nutrition, repeated frequently by the media, generated by different food and pharmaceutical industries. Thus, keep referring back to Perfect Self Control regularly to avoid any confusion in the future.

You only need to study the information directly relating to your particular blood group as descri-bed through Chapters 4-7 so that you take in only relevant information. Focus only on yourself. Once you feel confident applying the principles, it is best to start your diet with fruits next mor-ning based on the guidance in this program, but it is also possible to gradually change your ea-ting habits for a smoother transition. Of course, following the recommended diet strictly would be ideal; nevertheless, any steps towards the appropriate diet may significantly improve your health.

Due to our natural biorhythm, morning defecation is the healthiest. This can be strongly facilita-ted by consuming fruit for breakfast which cleanses the entire digestive system from the inside, pushing the remains of foodstuffs out of the stomach as well as any matter that may be stuck in the intestines. This may be unusual for you at the beginning, and you may feel that these morning fruits are causing diarrhea, but this is the first step to cleaning up our body. It only means that your natural biorhythm is returning while your body is detoxified. In a couple of days you will adapt to this, and return to normal bowel movements again. To avoid some unpleasant situations at the beginning, you may decide to start your new diet at the weekend or a holiday.

After consuming your first brunch or lunch, appropriately prepared from complex carbohydrates and vegetables, you will be astonished that the heavy, uneasy feelings, and the tiredness usually experienced after meals disappears. This perception is not due to unsuitable meals, but on the contrary, your stomach will not need to struggle as it did before because of the easier digestion. You will feel your stomach empty in three hours, since the food will be completely predigested by then and have passed through to the large intestine. It may be that you will feel hungry after eating this easily digested food, and you start to crave a quick and easy energy intake. But you should hold on and eat nothing, drinking water and tea instead until the next meal.

Since your body has not wasted energy on heavy digestion, it will spend its energy on the main problem, namely the detoxification of harmful acidic compounds stored in your tissues. First of all, your tissues will expel these toxins into your blood circulation. When these toxins reach your kidneys, they are filtered and emptied from your body through the urine. Don't worry if your urine has a strong smell for a couple of days, or if you experience headaches or nausea as these are the consequences of cleansing toxins from your body and any unpleasantness will be over before long.

You may find that your appetite is reduced too. In this case, you should slightly push yourself to eat a full meal, since the fruits, vegetables and fluids are there for you, helping to get rid of toxins released from your tissues. You can eat as much as 4-5 kg of fruit before noon.

In the afternoon, drinking 3-4-liters of mineral water or tea is advised and you should take long walks and go cycling, or do any physical exercise and enjoy a sauna to facilitate detoxification by sweating. Perspiration is especially important, as there are toxins that can be removed from our body only by sweating.

Your first dinner should consist of sea fish or poultry with vegetables, and take calcium and magnesium supplements before eating. 600-800 mg calcium and 200-300 mg magnesium are recommended, or rather the corresponding amount of complex bone-building supplement for good sleep at night. The first couple of days will be difficult, but you will soon adapt to your natural biorhythm, which your body has evolved to.

In 3-5 days, you will feel the positive effects of the Perfect Self Control system. Keep up with it! If you get through the first few days, you will feel better than ever before. You will be full of energy, your stamina and strength will increase, you will learn faster with increased memory capacity. Your eyesight and hearing will improve, while your skin will be smoother, and you will feel good. Furthermore, by being healthy, your ageing slows down, and some weeks later, you will forget the majority of diseases and sicknesses that you suffered from or were subject to.

Excess fat will slowly but surely disappear in a few months, and do not torture yourself to lose weight faster, as it may have a negative effect on your wellbeing. Always satisfy your appetite with appropriate meals at the right time. You will have more energy, thus you can gradually increase your physical exercises. Choose a hobby or sport and move as much as you wish to.

Instead of driving your car, you should walk or cycle, saving on fuel and protecting the environment. In a mid-sized town, in most cases bicycles are almost as fast as cars and you are spared the hassle of parking. In this way, you save time on exercise as well.

If you suffer from a serious disease, consult your doctor at the beginning of your new diet. For example, if you suffer with diabetes, injecting insulin when you follow your new diet may cause hypoglycemia, so the medication will need to be reduced over time. Moreover, if the diabetes is not too advanced, you may recover from it and restore the healthy working of your pancreas if you follow this diet.

Let me share with you some personal experiences. One of my distant relatives was diagnosed with metastatic breast cancer. Her physician prescribed a mastectomy as well as chemotherapy in three phases. Before her mastectomy I persuaded her to follow a diet according to her blood group A.

Between her mastectomy and the beginning of chemotherapy, her physician ordered further medical examinations to compare with previous results about the status of her cancer. Once the results were available, her physician called her in for consultation. She believed that the hour of her death was about to come, but the doctor cancelled the chemotherapy treatments, having found no metastatic tumors in her lungs, which had been there before the surgery. Thereafter the physician explained that her cancer was indeed in an advanced stage, that according to statistics, she had had approximately 1% chance of survival after the 3rd treatment of chemotherapy. But she recovered by changing to a healthy diet.

One of my friends, André Ortner who was a professional powerlifter, complained to me about his injured shoulder joints that forced him to give up on his training and competitions. He had sought out several medical experts, but they could not help him. I told him not to despair, suggesting a couple of specialized foods and nutritional supplements, which healed his shoulder joints. Following this, we had some great conversations about the importance of nutrition for sports. Thus, I convinced him to follow the appropriate diet. Subsequently, he won the world championship seven times in powerlifting, bench-pressing 372 kg, beating several records in his field.

The Effects and Characteristic Features of Foods

The following tables help you to find and learn the special effects and characteristics of different foods, and provide information on what foods require heat-treatment and which ones do not, for healthy digestion. If a maximum daily intake is indicated, please do not exceed it! Different foodstuffs contain a vast supply of fat-soluble vitamins or minerals and although they are vital for us, overdosing on these is terribly harmful and dangerous.

You will find an indicator number on a scale from -5 to +5, showing how useful or harmful the considered food is for your blood type. These numbers also show, if no maximum limit is defined, the proportional amount of recommended consumption:

+5	**is a basic nutrient, its daily intake is necessary**
+4	**is a basic nutrient, its regular intake is essential**
+3	**is very healthy**
+2	**is healthy**
+1	**is favorable**
0	**is neutral, but it is recommended to diversify your diet**
-1	**is unfavorable, but its occasional consumption is not really harmful**
-2	**is unhealthy, but its occasional consumption in small portions is not really harmful**
-3	**is considerably unhealthy, and it should be avoided**
-4	**is harmful, it must be avoided**
-5	**is very harmful, never consume it**

Some foods are especially effective to strengthen certain functions of our body and brain; these features are found in the appendix.

Fruits: Ripe and tasty fruit was the most important source of carbohydrate until the emergence of blood group A in plant-cultivating societies. But it is also important for people with type O and B blood. Before our ancestors climbed down from trees, it was the only source of carbohydrates. Fruit is the only food that our body does not have to break down to glucose, fructose and amino acids, since these are the basic elements of fruits with enzymes, vitamins, minerals and crystal-clear water. Each piece of fruit is a living thing, full of vital enzymes and vitamins, essential for health.

As soon as fruit is picked from the tree and cut, pushed, hit or heated, it begins to die, consequently vitamins and enzymes in it start decaying and decomposing very fast. Since cooking kills fruit at once together with its vital living enzymes and vitamins and makes it indigestible, we must always eat fruit on an empty stomach in a fresh and non-heat-treated state. If preferred, you can prepare fruit salads or smoothies, but always consume them immediately. Be aware not to chew fruit seeds, as they are oily seeds and digested as complex carbohydrates.

FRUITS	EFFECTS AND FEATURES	0	A	B	AB
Apple	contains plenty of roughage and amino acids; clears intestines	+5	+5	+5	+5
Apricot	contains plenty of carotene	0	+5	+2	+3
Banana	contains plenty of amino acids, potassium and magnesium; slightly alkaline when ripe and brown spots are on its surface	+5	0	+5	+2
Blueberry	contains plenty of carotene, but acidic	-4	+4	-1	1
Cherry	first fresh fruit of spring without high acid-content	0	+5	+3	+4
Currant	contains plenty of carotene, but acidic	-4	+2	-1	+1
Date	high-calorie food	+3	+1	+4	+2
Gooseberry	low energy supplier, but contains vital minerals	-2	+2	0	+1
Grape	contains elements essential for eyes and joints	+5	0	+5	+2
Kiwi	contains plenty of vitamin C, but acidic	-4	+3	0	+1
Mango	rich on minerals; protective effect on stomach	0	+1	+3	+2
Mulberry	contains plenty of carotene, but acidic	-3	+4	0	+2
Papaya	contains plenty of vitamin C and carotene	+1	-1	+4	+2
Peach	contains plenty of niacin	0	+2	+2	+2
Pear	excessive consumption may cause kidney stone	+3	0	+3	+1
Pineapple	contains enzymes that help losing weight	0	+4	+4	+4
Plum	helps with digestion and bowel movements	+4	3	+5	+4
Raspberry	contains plenty of carotene, but acidic	-4	+4	0	+2
Sour cherry	contains plenty of carotene, but acidic	+2	+3	+3	+3
Strawberry	contains plenty of vitamin C, but acidic	-4	+3	0	+2

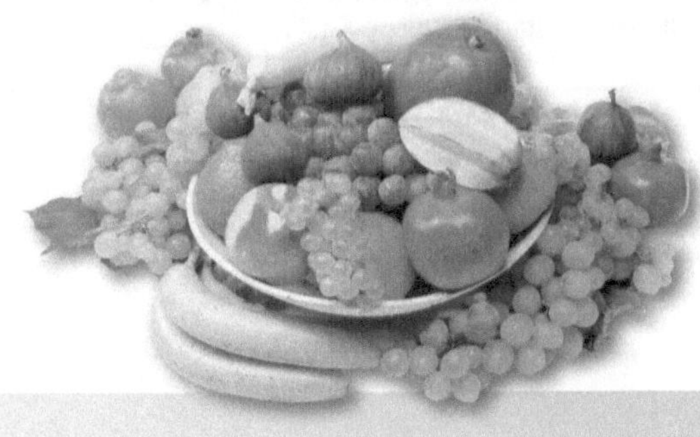

Citrus fruits

Although being acidic, they are not acidifying because from the human body citric acids evaporate through the skin.

CITRUS FRUITS	EFFECTS AND FEATURES	0	A	B	AB
Lemon	sour but not acidifying	0	+4	+5	+4
Lime	sour but not acidifying	-2	+1	+4	+2
Orange	sour but not acidifying	0	+1	+4	+3
Grapefruit	sour but not acidifying	-3	+4	+5	+4
Tangerine	sour but not acidifying	+1	+1	+4	+3

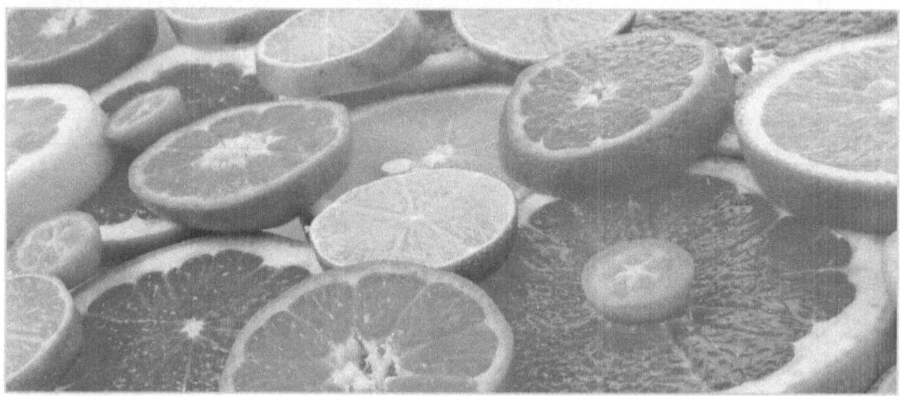

MELONS	EFFECTS AND FEATURES	0	A	B	AB
Honeydew melon	contains plenty of water and carotene	-1	+2	0	+1
Watermelon	contains plenty of water and carotene	-1	+2	0	+1

Watermelons and **honeydew melons** are actually cucurbitaceous plants (which includes plants like pumpkin and zucchini) but are digested as fruit.

	EFFECTS AND FEATURES	0	A	B	AB
Pepper	digestible as fruit as well as vegetable	-1	-1	+4	1
Tomato	digestible as fruit as well as vegetable	+4	-3	0	-1

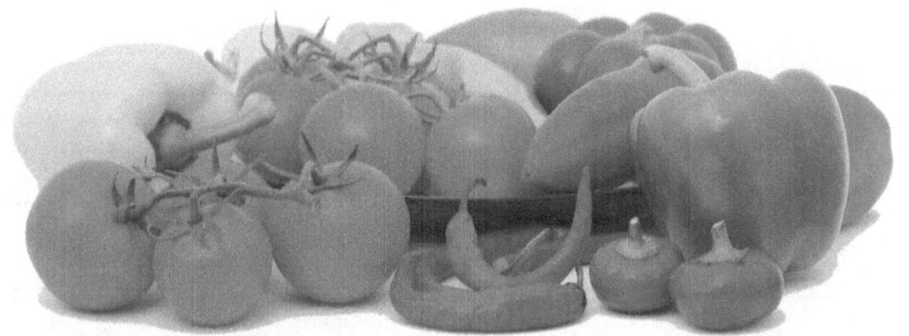

Peppers and **tomatoes** are somewhere between fruits and vegetables. They are digestible as fruit or as vegetable, but only in raw state.

Vegetables to be consumed in raw state:

EAT ROW!	EFFECTS AND FEATURES	0	A	B	AB
Cucumber	beautifies the skin	+4	+5	+4	+4
Black radish	cleans kidney and strongly alkalizing	+2	+2	0	+1
Cabbage	heavily digestible	-3	-2	+4	0
Lettuce	becomes bitter if exposed to irons	+1	+2	+1	+2
Radish	strongly alkalizing	+2	+2	0	+1

Bulbous vegetables like onion are digestible both in raw or heat-treated state. Each of them has an antibacterial and demulcent effect. **Raw garlic is the only plant on Earth, which has an additional antivirus effect, for this reason nowadays eating daily maximum 1-2 cloves of garlic and bulbous vegetables is important to preserve good health.** Exceeding the consumption of this amount of garlic must be avoided, since overdosing on some of its elements is very harmful.

	EFFECTS AND FEATURES	0	A	B	AB
Garlic	antibacterial and antiviral, prevents inflammations and irritations, protects us against cardiovascular diseases, cleans blood and veins; exceeding recommended consumption is hazardous. It causes hemophilia and other health issues. Max. 1-2 cloves per day.	+5	+5	+5	+5
Bulbous vegetables	antibacterial and prevent inflammations and irritations.	+5	+5	+5	+5

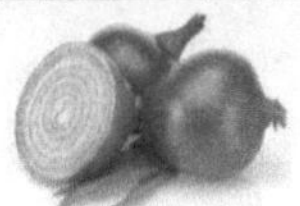
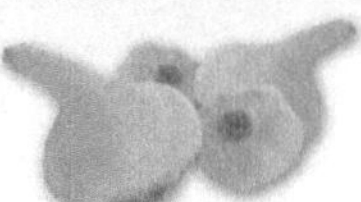
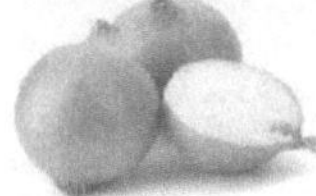

Vegetables what only digestible in cooked state:

COOK THESE!	EFFECTS AND FEATURES	0	A	B	AB
Asparagus	diuretic and clears kidney stone.	+2	+3	+2	+3
Beetroot	Contains plenty of carotene, thus limited intake is recommended	+4	+4	+4	+4
Broccoli	Contains plenty of amino acids and carotene.	+5	+3	+4	+4
Brussels sprout	Contains plenty of amino acids and vitamin K	-1	+3	+5	+5
Carrot	Contains plenty of carotene and amino acids, thus limiting intake is recommended	+4	+4	+4	+4
Cauliflower	Contains plenty of amino acids	-1	+4	+4	+4
Celery	aphrodisiac for men, increases sexual potency and the quantity of sperm	+4	+2	+4	+4
Ginger	Sooths inflammations and cramps, calms stomach and helps to lose weight; strongly aromatic	+4	+4	+4	+4
Ginkgo biloba	Improves cerebration.	+5	+5	+5	+5
Ginseng	Stimulates the brain, increases physical and sexual potency.	+4	+4	+4	+3
Horseradish	Effective against kidney and urinary tract infections, aromatic oils in fresh horseradish are antibacterial and clean respiratory system	+2	+4	+2	+3

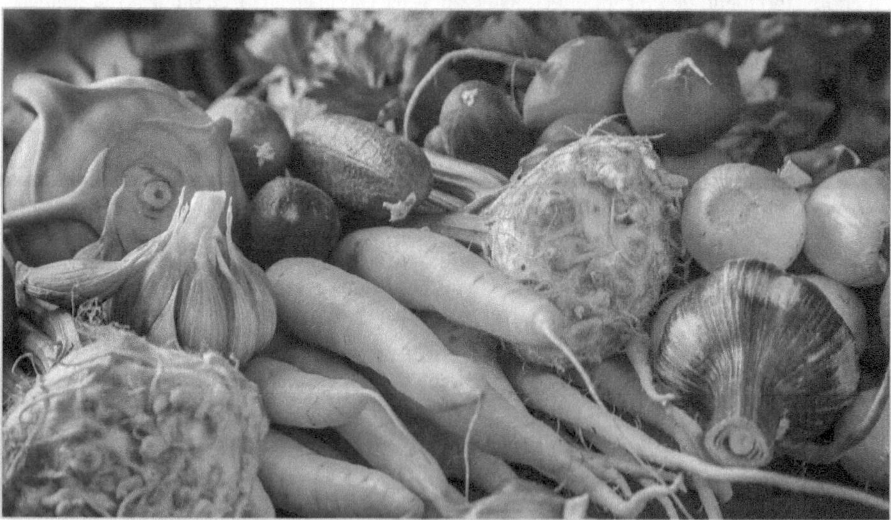

		0	A	B	AB
Kohlrabi	Contains plenty of vitamins	+4	+4	+3	+4
Olives	Max. 1-2 pieces per day, exceeding recommended amount is dangerous and carcinogenic!	-5	-2	-3	-2
Parsley	Contains plenty of amino acids	+4	+4	+4	+4
Sorrel	Contains plenty of iron and carotene	-1	+4	0	+2
Spinach	Contains plenty of iron and carotene	+4	+4	+2	+3

Complex carbohydrates: Each of the complex carbohydrates is predigested by the same alkaline digestive juice (according to the second digestion program) in approximately 3 hours.

Certain fruits and vegetables are only digestible as carbohydrate and indigestible with animal protein, since they belong rather to complex carbohydrates. For example, potato, pumpkin, zucchini, and eggplant are vegetable, however, due to their high content of starch or oil, they are digested as complex carbohydrates.

Fungi are closer to animals than to plants but actually belong to neither group, therefore they consist of complex proteins that are absolutely indigestible. Furthermore, each of them, even those that are called non-poisonous, contains an extremely high amount of toxins. For this reason, it is best to avoid their consumption. Never eat mushroom together with animal protein, because the easy digestion of animal protein would be impeded. Fig belongs to the fruits group, however, due to the small seeds inside, is digested as oily seeds. Hence it is recommended to consume them along with complex carbohydrates. Avocado is a special fruit, digested similarly to carbohydrates due to its high content of oil thus best eaten by itself.

	EFFECTS AND FEATURES	0	A	B	AB
Avocado	High content of oil, thus requires special digestion, eat only by itself	-4	+4	-4	0
Cucurbit	High content of starch, digested as complex carbohydrates	+2	+4	0	+2
Eggplant	High content of starch and oil, digested as complex carbohydrates	-1	-1	+3	+1
Fig	Eat it raw, digested as oily seeds due to tiny seeds inside	-4	+4	-3	0
Fungi	Indigestible (even in cooked state), high content of toxins never eat them with animal protein	-5	-5	-5	-5
Potato	High content of starch, digested as complex carbohydrates	+3	0	+3	+2
Pumpkin	High content of starch, digested as complex carbohydrates	+2	+4	1	+3
Zucchini	High content of starch and oil, digested as complex carbohydrates	0	+1	0	+1

The following grains after soaking in cereal form, are edible raw or in a cooked state, but only use their wholegrain version, as they contain vitamin B and essential fibers for the absorption of vitamin B. Both of them are necessary to base the proper environment in the colon for the digestion of the evening animal protein. Fibers and vitamin B are essential for our digestive system as well as for the healthy functioning of our brain and nervous system and humans can absorb them only from the whole grain. It is easier to digest them after cooking.

RAW OR COOKED	EFFECTS AND FEATURES	0	A	B	AB
Amaranth	high content of carbohydrates and starch	-1	+2	-1	+1
Barley	high content of carbohydrates and starch	-1	+2	0	+1
Oat	high content of carbohydrates and starch	+3	+4	+3	+4
Rye	high content of carbohydrates and starch	0	+1	0	+1
Wheat	high content of carbohydrates and starch	-5	+3	-3	+1

The following complex carbohydrates are edible only in cooked state:

COOK THESE!	EFFECTS AND FEATURES	0	A	B	AB
Brown rice	Contains fiber, vitamin B and amino acids, everything required for efficient digestive system	+4	+5	+4	+5
Buckwheat	high content of carbohydrates and starch	-1	+4	0	+2

PULSES	EFFECTS AND FEATURES	0	A	B	AB
Beans	High content of vegetable protein and phosphorus	-1	+2	0	+2
Corn	Only belongs to pulses due to its digestion, high content of carbohydrate	-5	+4	-3	0
Lentils	High content of vegetable protein and iron	-3	+4	-2	+1
Peas	High content of vegetable protein and calcium	0	+4	+1	+3

There are slight differences in the recommendation values between various types of peas, beans, and lentils, as the values above are understood in a general sense. Due to their high content of vegetable protein, pulses are not as easily digested as other complex carbohydrates.

Oily seeds: Oily seeds are complex carbohydrates, their digestion is independent of heat-treatment, but heating transforms the oil into trans-fat, thus the heat-treatment should be avoided.

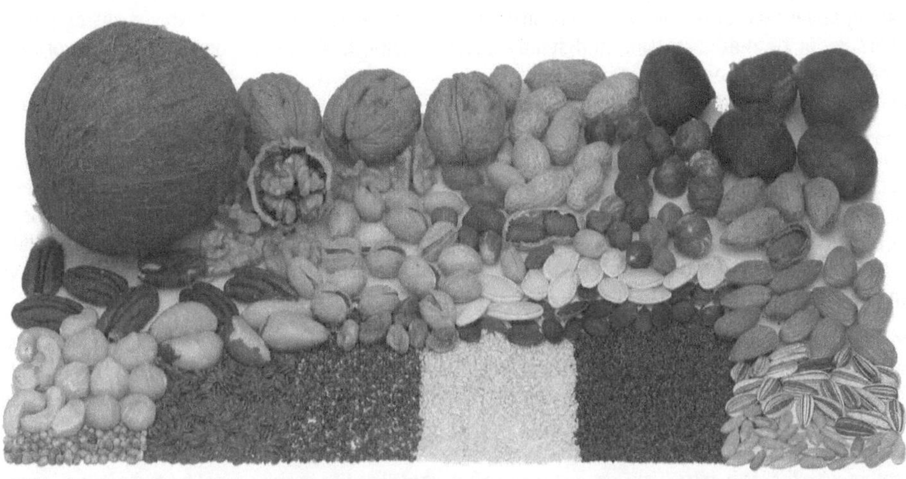

OILY SEEDS	EFFECTS AND FEATURES	0	A	B	AB
Almond	A couple of pieces per day has a beautifying effect on skin; high-calory food due to its high oil content	-1	+2	-1	+1
Walnuts	High-calory food due to its high oil content	-1	+2	-1	+1
Hazel	High-calory food due to its high oil content	-5	+4	-5	-1
Sunflower seed	High-calory food due to its high oil content	-5	+2	-4	0
Pumpkin seed	High-calory food due to its high oil content	-1	+5	-1	+1
Pistachio	High-calory food due to its high oil content	-2	+1	-1	+1
Sesame	High-calory food due to its high oil content	-3	+3	-3	0
Chestnut	High-calory food due to its high oil content	-3	+2	-3	0
Poppy	High-calory food due to its high oil content	-3	+2	-3	0
Coconut	High-calory food due to its high oil content	-1	+3	-1	+1
Peanut	High-calory food due to its high oil content	-2	+3	-2	0
Mustard	High-calory food due to its high oil content	-2	+4	-2	+1
Cashew	High-calory food due to its high oil content	-2	+1	-2	0
Cocoa	Its minerals and vasodilating effect are beneficial for the brain, and help to prevent cardiovascular diseases	+2	+5	+3	+4

Taking advantage of our instinctive desire for **cocoa** products, the food industry earns billions of dollars profit by manufacturing and selling chocolate. Its flavor should be derived from original cocoa. However, it is an expensive ingredient.

Chocolate was originally made from cocoa beans by the Aztecs. Nowadays the majority of chocolates are made from cheap, hydrogenated vegetable oils, with synthetic flavorings, sugar and milk powder. These synthetic substances provide a stronger and tastier flavoring than cocoa, but these are carcinogenic chemicals. Cocoa butter may be added to these products, but it is only the fat of cocoa, which is likewise unhealthy. High-quality chocolates usually contain a certain amount of cocoa, but most chocolates - unlike traditional cocoa - are usually very harmful. Cocoa gives an excellent flavor to our desserts and sweets, and if we consume traditional cocoa made from cocoa beans, we can enjoy its beneficial effects.

The preparation of animal protein with some expectations always requires heat-treatment. Every type of meat or fish consists of different very complex chains of proteins. Every kind of animals needs different types of acidic digestive enzymes to break down. For this reason, simultaneous digestion of different animal protein types is impossible. The most complex proteins are found in mammalian meat. Poultry proteins are les complex, fish proteins are simpler. Egg and dairy products are the simplest, so they can be consumed and digested together with fish or poultry; however, meat and offal, as well as fish have to come from the same species for the easy and perfect digestion. The blood very fast gets off after the death of the animal and full of toxin so try to reduce its consumption as much as possible by socking the meat or fish in could salty water.

Meat for mammals:

RED MEATS	EFFECTS AND FEATURES	0	A	B	AB
Beef	High content of iron	+3	-3	+5	+1
Lamb	High content of iron	+3	-3	+5	+1
Goat meat	High content of iron	+3	-3	+5	+1
Their liver	High content of toxins and fat-soluble vitamins	+1	-5	+4	-2

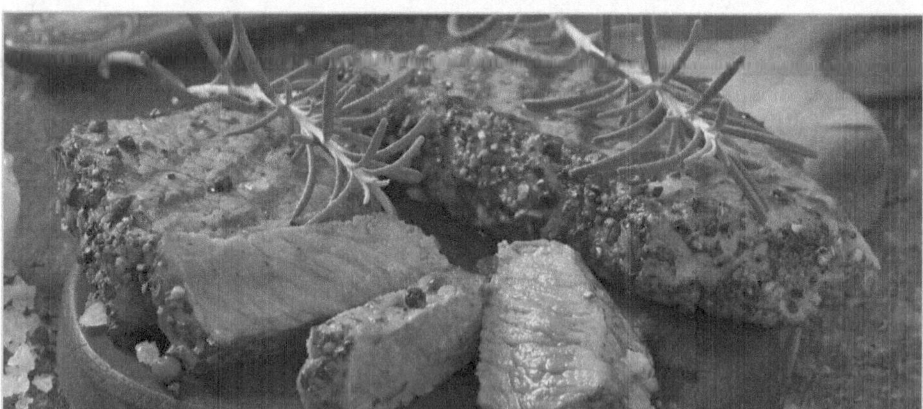

ACIDIC RED MEATS WITH TAPEWORMS	EFFECTS AND FEATURES	0	A	B	AB
Rabbit	Acidifying; high content of uric acids and toxins due to tapeworms living in them	-5	-5	-5	-5
Pork	Acidifying; high content of uric acids and toxins due to tapeworms living in them	-5	-5	-5	-5
Boar	Acidifying; high content of uric acids and toxins due to tapeworms living in them	-5	-5	-5	-5

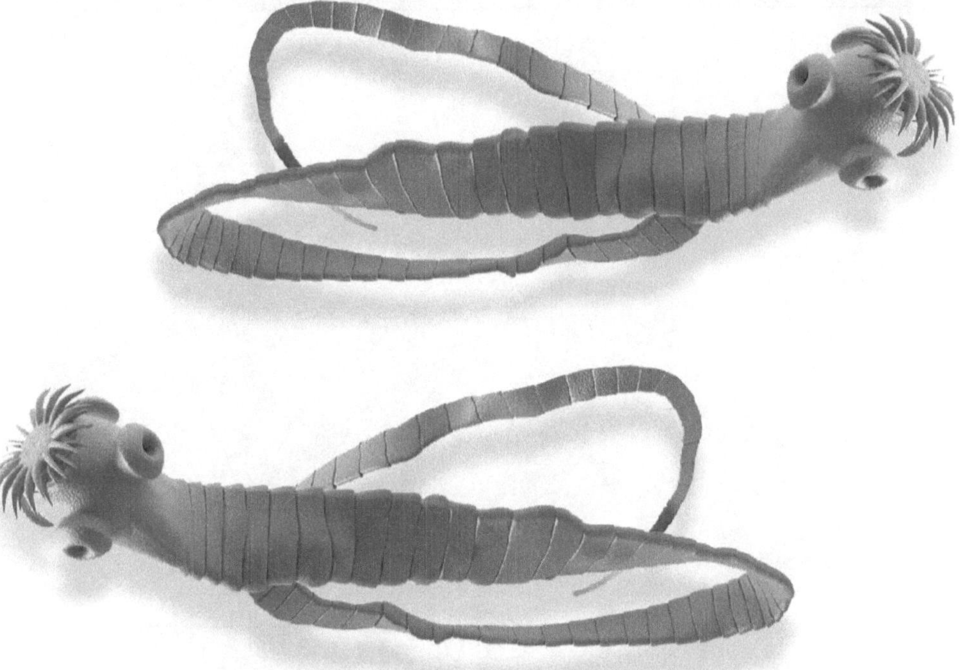

Avoid eating meat such as pork, which is consumed by tapeworms what defecate strongly acidic, toxic excrement into the flesh of pig. Thanks to the feces of these worms, pork and these kinds of meat are extremely acidifying because of uric acid and toxins. Therefore, these animals are not really adequate for human consumption. Eating their raw meat infects us with these worms.

POULTRY	EFFECTS AND FEATURES	0	A	B	AB
Chicken	Unfavorable due to its mineral content	+3	+1	-5	-3
Turkey	Favorable due to amino acids and minerals	+3	0	-2	-2
Duck	Its meat is fatty	+4	-2	-2	-2
Goose	Its meat is fatty	+5	+2	+1	+3
Ostrich	Its meat is dry and hard to chew	+3	-2	-2	-2
Their liver	High content of toxins and fat-soluble vitamins, thus eat with moderation; chicken liver should not be consumed by blood group B and AB individuals	+3	-3	+1	-1

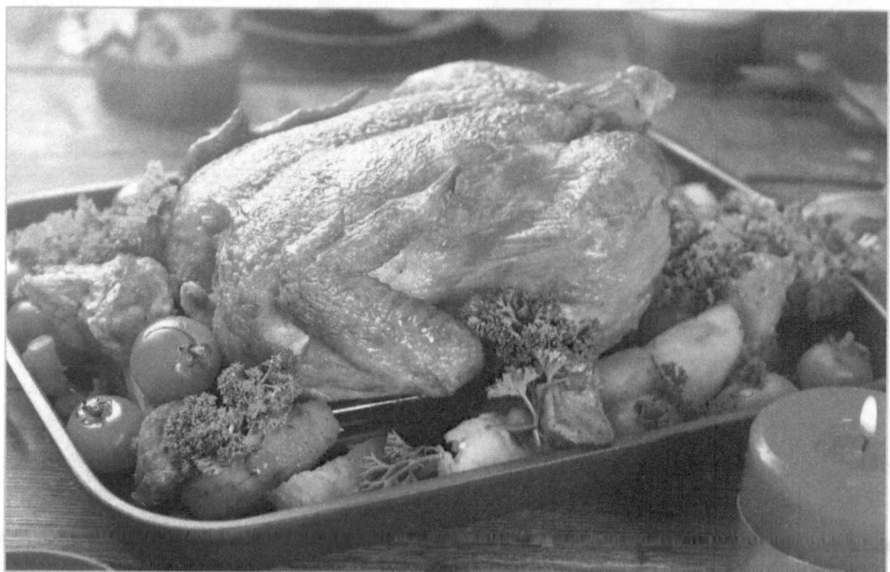

	EFFECTS AND FEATURES	0	A	B	AB
Egg	High content of cholesterol, minerals, and fat-soluble vitamins, without containing loads of toxin	+5	-1	+3	+1

Egg has to be heat-treated due to the salmonella bacteria in it, but if its yolk hardens too much, it will be hardly digestible. For this reason, soft-boiled egg is recommended, or if you prepare Sunnyside-up egg, fry it only until the white part is hard, but the yolk is still soft. Salmonella already perishes on 80 °C / 170 °F.

Sea food:

Deep-sea fish especially have a really positive effect on the functions of our brain and our nerves, blood circulation and on our whole body altogether, due to the omega 3 and omega 6 unsaturated fatty acids and fat-soluble vitamins contained in it. These nutrients are essential for everyone. Without the addition of deep-sea fish into the diet, the brain and nervous system cannot function satisfactorily, thus we will be subject to psychological and nervous system diseases. Unsaturated fatty acids contained in plants are only similar to those contained in sea fish, our brain cannot use them.

AQUATIC ANIMALS	EFFECTS AND FEATURES	0	A	B	AB
Scaly sea fish	The oldest and only source of omega 3 and omega-6 unsaturated fatty acids, fat-soluble vitamins, protein; these are essential for our brain and nervous system; consume sea-fish for dinner at least 3 times a week	+5	+4	+4	+4
Aquatic animals without scale	As these animals are necrophagous (eating dead animals) or apex predators, they contain high amount of toxins and undesired proteins, hence they are carcinogenic	-4	-5	-5	-5

Unfortunately, the oceans are extremely polluted. They are full of poisons such as PCBs, or polychlorinated biphenyls, (industrial products or chemicals) which cannot be eliminated from living beings, but these toxins are stored in fatty tissues. When sea predators eat another aquatic animal, these poisons are consumed and stored in their fatty tissues. This is the reason why predators at the top of a food chain and necrophagous animals - those that feed on dead animals - accumulate the highest amount of toxins.

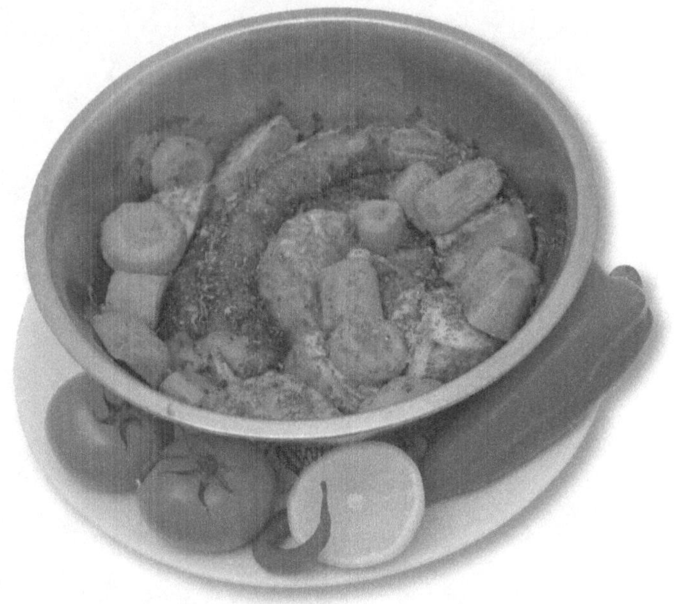

We do not need to be concerned about the heat-treatment of **milk and dairy products**, since only pasteurized products may be sold.

DAIRY PRODUCTS	EFFECTS AND FEATURES	0	A	B	AB
Cow milk	High content of calcium, lactose, and fat-soluble vitamins	-5	-3	+4	+1
Sour yogurt	High content of calcium and fat-soluble vitamins, barely and content of lactose	-1	0	+5	+4
Yogurt	High content of calcium and fat-soluble vitamins, low content of lactose	-2	-1	+5	+2
Goat milk	High content of calcium, lactose and fat-soluble vitamins	-5	-3	+4	0
Goat cheese	High content of calcium and fat-soluble vitamins, low content of lactose	-4	-2	+4	+1
Cottage cheese	High content of calcium and fat-soluble vitamins, low content of lactose	-3	-1	+4	+2

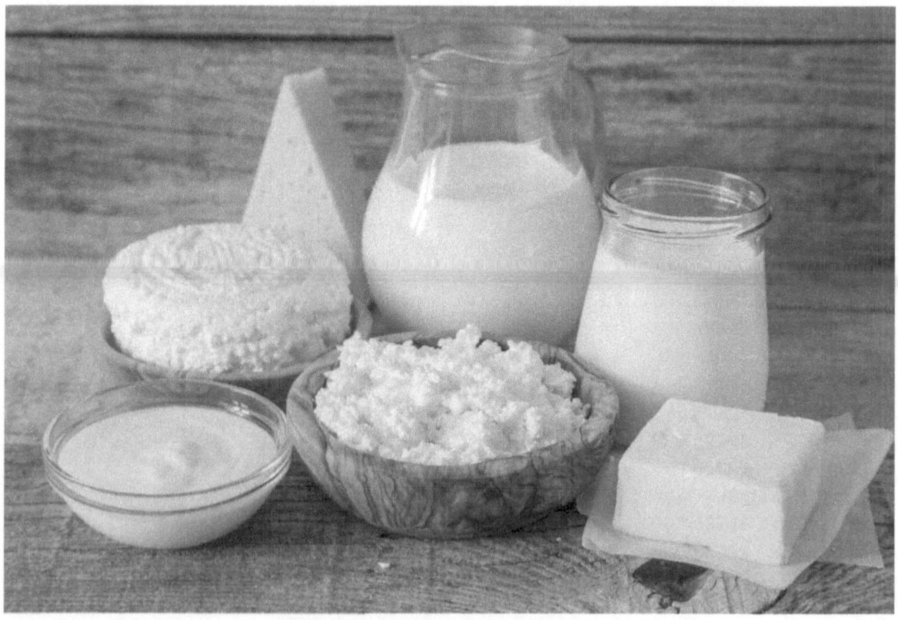

Cheeses: There are three basic groups of cheeses:

1. High quality cheeses with high content of calcium, and low content of sodium and fat. Usually they are yellow with holes in them. Includes: edam and emmental cheese, port salut.

2. Lower quality cheeses, with low content of calcium, and high content of sodium and fat. Usually they are white or light colored. Includes: cheeses in bulk, teddy cheese, mozzarella.

3. Blue or moldy cheeses, whose mold may be called noble mold, but these are types of mold without bad taste. These are poisonous fungi, producing strong toxins what are strongly carcinogenic, acidic and seriously harm the liver. These cheeses are very hazardous.

CHEESES	EFFECTS AND FEATURES	0	A	B	AB
High quality cheeses	High content of calcium and minerals, low content of lactose	-2	-1	+4	+1
Lower quality cheeses	Low content of minerals and protein, fattening due to high content of fats	-5	-4	-2	-3
Blue or moldy cheeses	Strongly carcinogenic and acidifying due to its high content of toxins	-5	-5	-5	-5

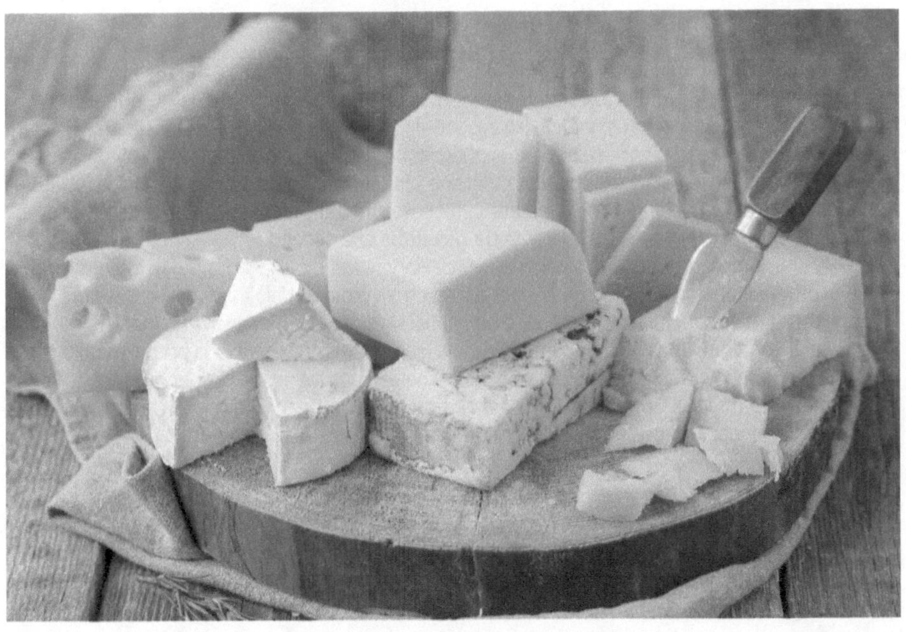

SWEETENERS	EFFECTS AND FEATURES	0	A	B	AB
Honey	Helps to heal wounds and injuries; high content of enzyme and vitamins, recommended upper limit per day is two tablespoons; contains only glucose and fructose, thus consumable by diabetics; since it is expensive, sugar and synthetic materials are often added, which crystalizes it after a while	0	+3	+2	+3
Sugar, brown sugar, cane sugar	Empty carbohydrate, fattening, increases the likelihood of diabetes, but not carcinogenic	-5	-1	-3	-1
Stevia	Completely natural with 0 calorie; has a slight aftertaste that is harmonized with the taste of coffee and tea; it is not fattening, acidifying, and carcinogenic	0	0	0	0
Eritril	Completely natural, thus not carcinogenic	-1	-1	-1	-1
Aspartam	Acidifying, controversial on carcinogenicity	-2	-4	-2	-3
Natrium cyclamate	Strongly acidifying and probably carcinogenic	-3	-5	-4	-5
Xylitol	High energy content and can cause diarrhea	-3	-1	-2	-1

Synthetic vitamin pills and drinks:

  Multivitamin commercials effectively mislead people to the idea that all the essential vitamins can be supplied by pills and drink supplements. The truth is that more than 200 different types of vitamins have been identified which are essential for healthy bodily functions and freely available in the food we eat. What's more, experts estimate the number of vitamins may be as many as 2000, but their chemical composition cannot be identified. This is because the real vitamins in fresh food are living compounds, and are subject to constant biochemical processes, thereby their constitution changes continuously in thousandths of a second.

Pills only contain synthetic, dead vitamins, which only resemble the genuine, living ones. From these synthetic substances, we can expect as much as from a visit to Madame Tussaud's waxworks museum and try to listen to how the wax version of Luciano Pavarotti sings.

Of course, if someone does not consume vitamins from fresh food at all, it is better to take these pills. But if you follow the Perfect Self Control diet, your body gains the proper amount and type of vitamins and minerals - no more, no less. If you follow a healthy diet, you should not take additional vitamins. And this applies to any other nutrients as well.

STIMULANT DRINKS	EFFECTS AND FEATURES	O	A	B	AB
Green tea	The healthiest stimulant drink; its effect lasts approximately 8 hours	+5	+2	+4	+3
Black tea	Black tea is the slightly rotten version of green tea, thus it is more acidifying; its effect lasts for approximately 4 hours	+3	+2	+2	+2
Chamomile tea	disinfectant, anti-inflammatory	0	0	0	0
Coffee	Only drink traditionally brewed coffee, never the instant version; although their taste is similar, traditional coffee is healthy for blood group A and AB individuals, while instant coffee is extremely acidifying and carcinogenic; its effect lasts for approximately 4 hours	-5	+4	-1	+2

Tap water:

If you use tap water, drink and cook only with cold water, as algae and fungi living in warm water tubes make warm tap water highly toxic. Moreover, you should rather avoid absolutely the consumption of any tap water, if it contains fluoride.

ALCOHOLIC BEVERAGES	EFFECTS AND FEATURES	O	A	B	AB
Beer	Alcohol destroys living tissues	-5	-1	-4	-2
Wine	Alcohol destroys living tissues	-1	-1	-1	-1
Hard liquor	Alcohol destroys living tissues	-5	-5	-5	-5

Alcohol

Alcohol dissolves living tissues, starting with the cell membrane. Since the cell membrane of our nervous and brain cells are the thinnest, enabling them to conduct electric signals, alcohol dissolves them first. When our brain and nervous cells are dying, we feel dizziness. Moreover, alcohol is the highest calorie carbohydrate with a serious fattening effect, catalyzing the development of type 2 diabetes. Thus, it is best to avoid alcohol consumption even in small quantities. Nevertheless, some glasses of wine or beer will not harm you seriously, as they contain less alcohol and toxins than hard liquors which should be avoided.

The tables above are valid in a general sense; small deviations for different individuals are possible, based on genes unrelated to blood groups or disabilities due to former diseases or injuries. Furthermore, it is incredibly important to consume dishes according to the Perfect Self Control system at the appropriate time of day, since for example, a highly recommended meat (+5) if consumed for breakfast without eating meat at night, is much worse for you than a non- recommended meat (-2) eaten at the right time for dinner.

Recipes:

1- Salads and Dressings

The base of every dressing is identical.
The following quantities are measured for one person.
Dressing base
- Freshly squeezed juice of half a lemon,
- 1 sweetener tablet
- pinch of black pepper
- pinch of sea salt
- Possibly 1-2 garlic cloves, finely chopped or crushed
- Possibly half an onion, chopped
- spices, suited to the type of salad.

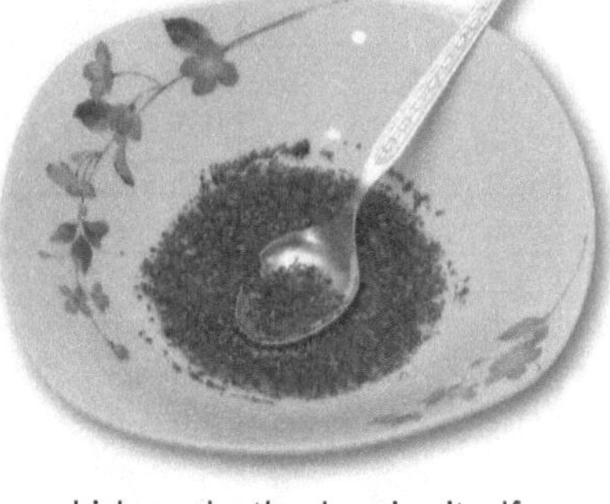

Mix the ingredients above together to get the dressing base which can be the dressing itself.
Salads:

If you prefer dairy-based dressings, stir the dressing base into 200-300 ml / 7-10 fl oz of dairy products (as suited to your blood group) or into soya yogurt. Then mix the dressing or just the dressing base with the chopped vegetables, and the salad is ready.

A wide variety of salads can be prepared from our favorite vegetables. We should try to choose fresh, ripe, and good-quality vegetables, since the flavor of any dish is mostly determined by the taste of ingredients used for the preparation. For example, if you have a cucumber that is already sour, it is best thrown away instead of using it up and spoiling the taste of the entire meal. It is essential to find the most appropriate sources of good-quality and tasty food and ingredients.

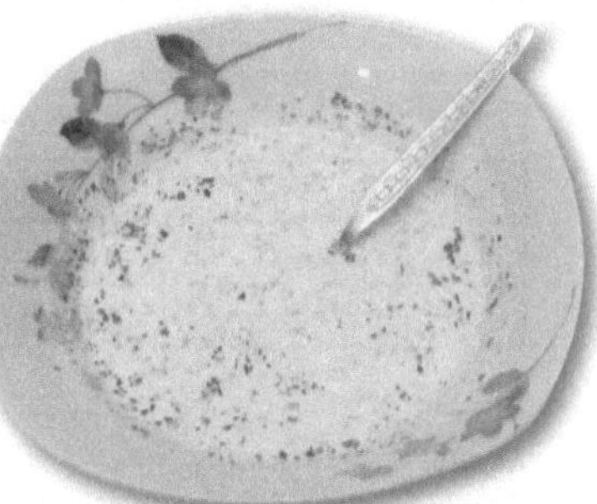

These salads are basically separated into three groups in terms of their dressing:

A. Dairy dressing
The dressing of the first group is prepared from dairy products added to the dressing base.
-     Blood group O should only use sour yogurt
-     Blood group A may use other yogurts
-     Blood groups B and AB may use all kinds of dairy products

It is important to buy good-quality, thick sour yogurt, which will give the dressing a more substantial base. We may consume these salads for dinner with poultry or fish dishes.

B. Soya and mustard dressing
The dressing of the second group is made from soya yogurt and possibly mustard added to the dressing base. We may eat these salads with complex carbohydrates.

C. Vegetable dressing
The third group of salads is prepared from tomato and other vegetables added to the dressing

base. We may dine on these salads with any meat or fish or complex carbohydrates; people with blood type A and AB should substitute bell pepper for tomato in these salads.

D. Herbs – Basil gives great flavor, especially to tomato and to any other vegetable. Oregano or dill and other herbs or spices also can be used to season the dressing to taste. If lettuce is used, be careful not to prepare it using metal cutlery or utensils. Contact with a metal surface makes the taste of lettuce unpleasantly bitter. You should use a ceramic or a glass bowl, and plastic or ceramic cutlery for its preparation and consumption. You can tear lettuce by hand, and slice other vegetables with a knife, but a plastic spoon is needed, at least for the final stage of the preparation.

Some suggestions for the seasoning of a healthy, traditional salad dressing.

Greek salad dressing

2 tea spoons of basil and 1 tea spoon of oregano. Mix the herbs into the base described above. Blood group A and AB individuals should add some extra virgin olive oil to the dressing.

This is also delicious with dairy products, but then it is no longer called a Greek salad unless you use a Greek cheese. For example, adding sour yogurt, sour cream, or yogurt is an excellent flavoring for the salad.

Thousand island salad dressing

Based on your preferences, you should add paprika, chili, and 2 dl / 7 fl oz sour yogurt and 1 dl sour cream to the base dressing. Based on your preferences, add the spices to taste, and the dairy products to the base dressing, and mix them.

Dill salad dressing

You should add some finely diced dill to the dressing base, then mix in 2-3 dl / 7-10 fl oz of sour yogurt, natural yogurt, or sour cream. Basil could also be added to the dressing base for a richer flavor, then mix in.

Basil salad dressing

1 table spoon of good quality basil should be added to the dressing base. Add fresh, well-washed, finely-chopped basil to the dressing base.

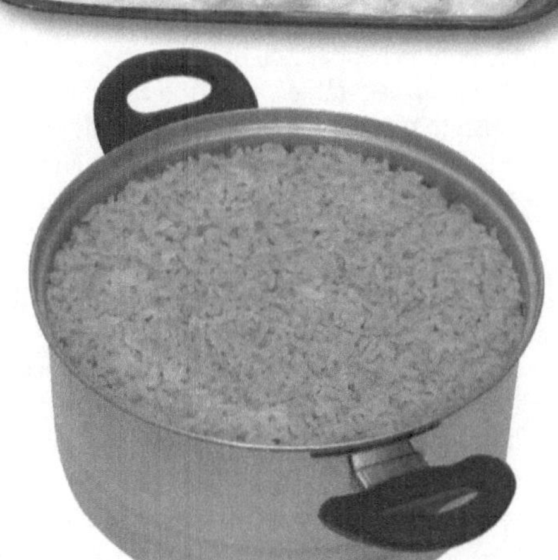

2- Using brown rice

Brown rice can be bought in ready-cooked form or in packet mixes, and in its normal dried state. It is better to buy the normal version as it is more likely that important nutrients of rice will be contained in it. Blood group A and AB individuals can cook it in the traditional way. After the rice is rinsed using a strainer and left to drain, sauté the rice in a little oil, add salt and then add boiling water to cover the rice two times higher than the level of rice. Cook on a low heat for approximately 70 minutes.

Blood group O and B individuals should not use oil for its preparation, therefore it is recommended to use a special rice-cooking pot. Use an electric stove with low heating if possible, gas stoves should be used with a metal trivet placed under the pot to reduce the heat. Thick-bottomed saucepans should be used for cooking in order to prevent burning if no fat or oil is added. Alternatively, you could spread some oil in your pan and heat it into its surface, then wipe down the oil with a paper towel, thereby avoiding subsequent burning without adding oil directly to the rice.

Due to its starch content, rice usually foams after twenty minutes of cooking, therefore remove the lid to keep from boiling over. If this happens, add water to refill the pot with water. However, if you wish to spare yourself the trouble, packet brown rice is easy to cook.

3- Seed shake

 Oily seeds suitable for our blood group should be blended together, flavored by milled cocoa, and mixed with honey. The resulting cream is more delicious than Nutella or any type of artificial nut cream. Furthermore, it is definitely healthy as it is made from oily seeds and honey, unlike their artificial version made of hydrogenated rape oil, sugar, artificial aromas and other additives. It is edible for a while, without adding any artificial additives. It is an excellent deli with Graham baps or pancakes.

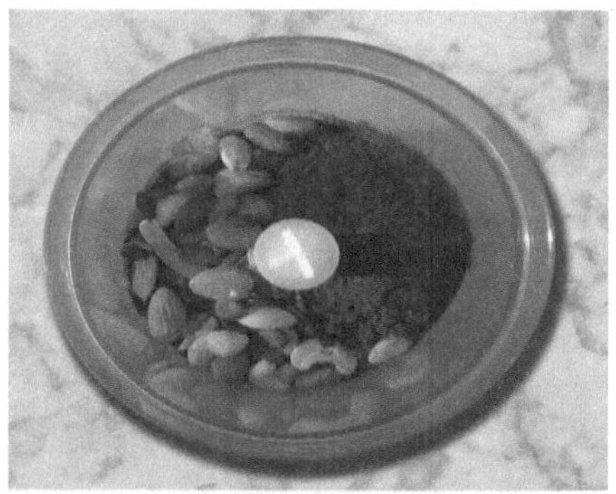 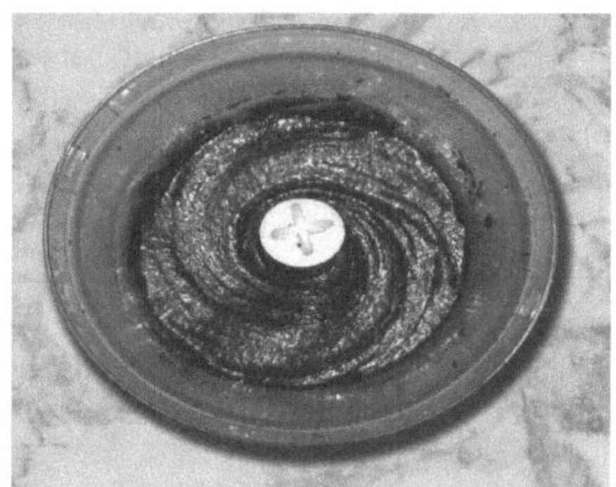

4- Breaded Fried Vegetables

- 0.6 liter / 1 pint of warm water (appr. 60-70°C / 140-160 F)
- as much oat flour as results in a dense paste
- 2 tablespoonfuls of corn or tapioca starch
- a teaspoon of salt
- chili, ground pepper and basil to taste

For breading vegetables, pour the warm water into a bowl, depending on the amount of vegetables you wish to prepare. (You can make it without measuring the temperature if you add 0.1 liter / 3,4 fl oz of cold water to 0.5 liter / 1 pint of boiling water). Stir in the oat flour to make it a thick paste, and the corn or tapioca starch, the salt, the chili, the ground pepper and the basil, then mix well. Leave for a couple of hours and stir again. If it is too thick, add some water, if it is too liquid, add some oat flour. Once it is ready, add any washed and sliced vegetables to your taste such as broccoli, cauliflower, zucchini, eggplant, or Brussels sprouts. You will need an oven with air circulation function, and always use baking paper on the ovens tray. After dipping the vegetables in the breading sauce, allow the sauce to drip off, and then roll them in bread crumbs to coat. Then put them trays covered with baking papers in a preheated oven (about 220°C / 420°F, at the strongest air circulation) and leave to cook for 40 minutes. Turn the vegetables

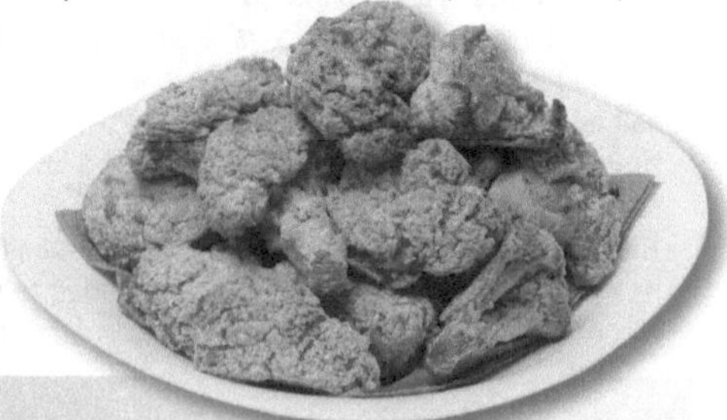

over after 20 minutes. This food is made without oil or eggs. Blood group A and AB individuals could use olive oil for frying if weight gain is no issue.

5-Vegan tartar sauce
- freshly squeezed juice of a quarter of a lemon
- 1-2 teaspoons of sugar (or 2-4 sweetener tablets)
- pinch of black pepper
- pinch of sea salt
- 2 tablespoons of strong mustard
- 300-400 ml / 10-13 fl oz soy yogurt

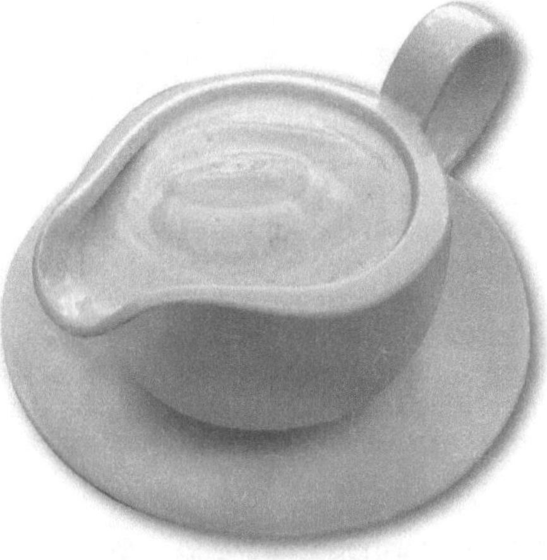

The above quantities are measured for one person. Mix all the ingredients well together.

You might add some garlic and basil for extra flavoring. The resulting vegan tartar sauce is delicious with breaded vegetables and an excellent supplement for mayonnaise in vegan salads with corn, peas or potato.Vegan tartar sauce is digested as complex carbohydrate due to its soy and mustard content. So, consume it with other complex carbohydrates and vegetables, never with animal protein.

6- Potato salad
Cook potatoes in their skin, then rinse in cold water, this makes peeling much easier. Furthermore, important nutriments are preserved.

Slice or dice the potato and add some sliced raw onion (about 1/3 the amount of potato), then add a little salt and black pepper then mix together with plenty of vegan tartar sauce.

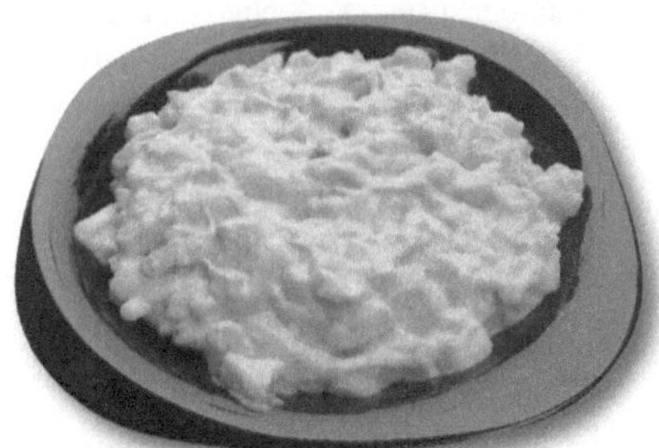

7- Vegetables Boiled in their Skin
Similar to cooking potatoes, stew vegetables in their skin and pour cold water on them to make peeling easier (in some cases you can pull off the whole skin at once) and important nutriments are saved by this.

The resulting vegetables are excellent for salad preparation or for a side dish with your dinner.

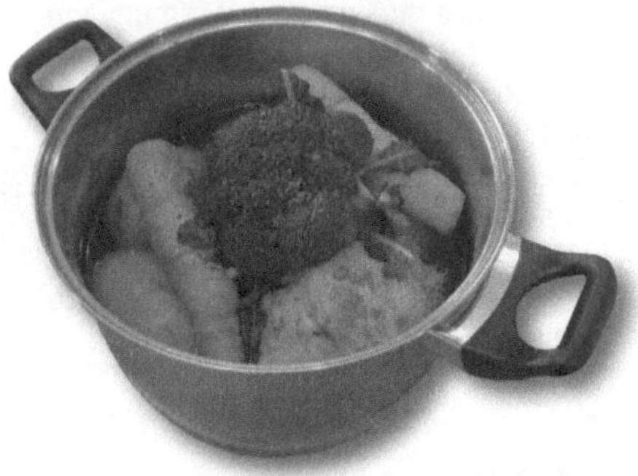

8- Frying Meat in a Ceramic Pan

Ceramic, unlike Teflon, is not carcinogenic. Use plastic or wooden kitchen spoons and utensils and a thick-bottomed high-quality ceramic frying pan which is large enough to fry everything at once.

Place it on the largest burner in order to receive sufficient heat to the sides of the pan to make its surface evenly hot. Before seasoning, you should cut the fat off the meat, and melt it in the pan at a low temperature, heating it up slowly. Remove any remaining pieces of meat from the fat, then heat it and make sure it covers the entire surface of the pan. Then you can wipe the fat off the pan with a paper towel, and then when you cook the meat, it will not stick to the surface and burn. However, if weight gain is not an issue, you do not need to bother with this. Be careful not to burn the fat and always wash your frying pan thoroughly.

For frying poultry, you may use duck or goose fat, or butter. You can also fry eggs in this way.

You should fry fish in its own fat and in the case of fatty fish, heat it up slowly, otherwise use butter or cod liver oil. Blood group A and AB individuals may use extra virgin olive oil as well.

Poultry and fish are delicious with the following flavorings: sea salt, pepper, chili, garlic, onion and any Mediterranean spice mix to taste. Also, herbs like rosemary, thyme, basil, oregano, and peppergrass suit fish and poultry well. Using too many spices simultaneously affects the taste of a dish negatively. Usually frying needs a preheated frying pan, or you can roast in the oven which is a little easier.

9- Ceramic Pan-Frying Fish or Chicken Breast Fillet

Slice fish fillet or chicken breast to half an inch thick and add the spices. (See recipes in Section 8.) Brown each side of the fish or chicken at a high temperature, then reduce the heat, cover the thick-bottomed ceramic frying pan and braise; chicken for 30-40 minutes, fish will need less time, about 20-40 minutes. A little boiling water may be added.

10-Ceramic pan-Frying turkey breast

Slice the turkey breast to half an inch thick, and season. (Recipes 8) Slightly brown one side of the sliced meat at a high temperature for about one minute, then reduce the heat to a minimum and fry for a further two minutes. Then turn the slices over and repeat the quick-frying followed by the gentle frying on the other side. You should fry turkey breast for no longer than 5-7 minutes, as in this way it becomes delicious. If you fry it for longer, it becomes hard and difficult to chew.

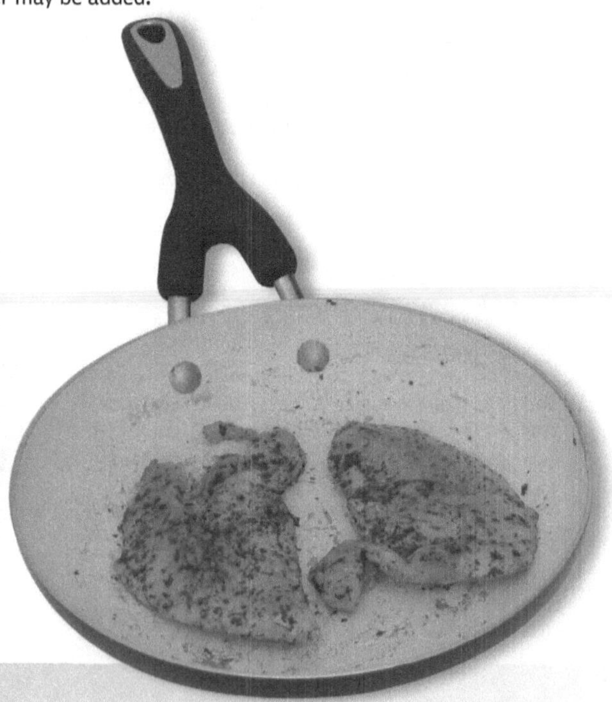

11- Dietary Duck Roasting

First, try to cut off the fat from the duck using a sharp knife. Then melt this fat in a ceramic frying pan at a low temperature. Leave the thigh, breast, back and offal (liver, gizzard, heart) in one piece, and season them to taste. For example, Provençal herb mix, chili, black pepper, finely-chopped garlic, and iodinated sea salt are excellent flavoring for duck. (Do not add salt to liver.) Remove any remaining lumps from the fat, and brown the duck at a high temperature for 10-15 minutes in the preheated frying pan. Then lift the parts of the duck from the pan and place on a paper towel to absorb the excess fat. Sprinkle some finely-chopped garlic and chili over the duck and place it into a casserole. Vegetables that require cooking may be added such as carrot, parsnip, celery, beetroot and onion. If no vegetables are added, pour some water into the casserole under the duck, place in the preheated moderately hot oven (180-200°C / 350-390°F) and roast for 120-180 minutes. You can serve duck with salad, roast vegetables and fried egg.

12- Ceramic Pan-Frying Steak

Steak may be fried in beef fat or even poultry fat or virgin olive oil. It should be flavored with sea salt, black pepper, chili, marjoram, and garlic to taste. (See recipes 8.) Rib eye steak takes approximately 7-12 minutes on a medium heat; sirloin steak, tenderloin steak, and rump steak take 10-16 minutes. Iron stake takes 12-15 minutes on a medium heat.

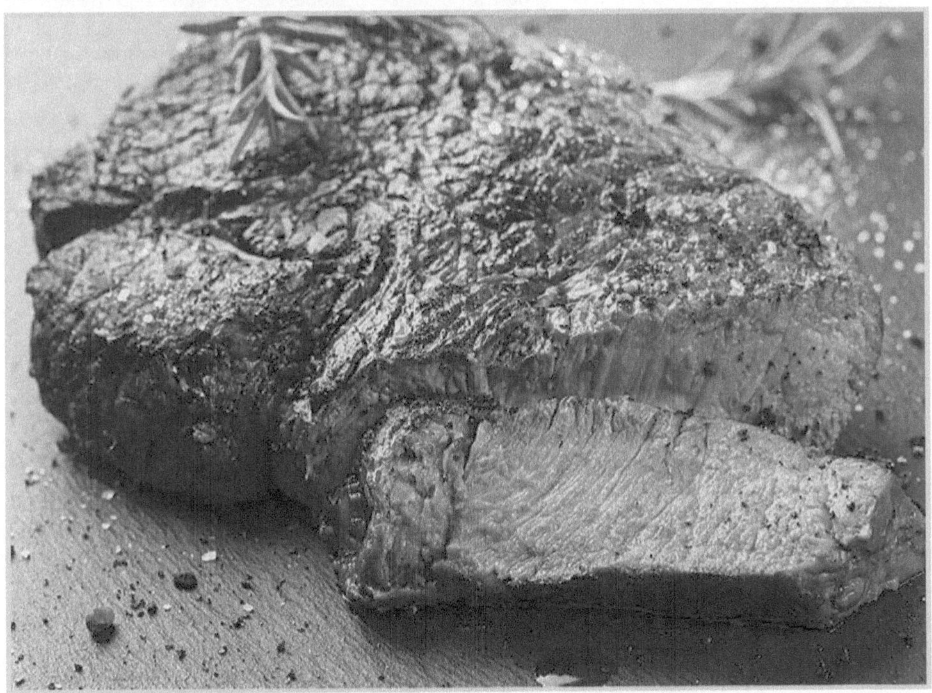

13-Ceramic Pan-Frying liver

With liver you should never add salt before cooking since salting it beforehand makes it tough and hard to chew. The best way to cook liver is to leave it in one piece without dicing. First leave it to soak in cold water for a few hours, then push or cut out the blood, wash thoroughly then spice it with black pepper, marjoram and garlic to taste. It is possible to roast liver together with meat in the oven. Alternatively, you may melt enough duck or goose fat to cover the liver in a smaller ceramic frying pan and fry the liver gently for 15 minutes. Then leave it on a paper towel to absorb the excess fat off the liver, and salt it.

14-Roasting in the Oven

First, gut and clean the meat or fish, then leave it to soak in cold salted water. Poultry and fish are delicious with the following flavorings: sea salt, pepper, chili, garlic, onion and Provençal or Italian, or Greek spice mixes to taste. Also, rosemary, thyme, basil, oregano, and peppergrass suit fish and poultry well. Using too many spices simultaneously, affects the taste of dish negatively.

Place the meat or fish into a roasting pan with some vegetables that require heat-treatment: carrots, parsnips, celery, beetroot, etc. Then cover the roasting pan and place in the oven to roast for the required time. For the last 10 minutes of cooking time, you can remove the lid to brown the meat or fish slightly. This is the most simple and practical way to cook animal protein.

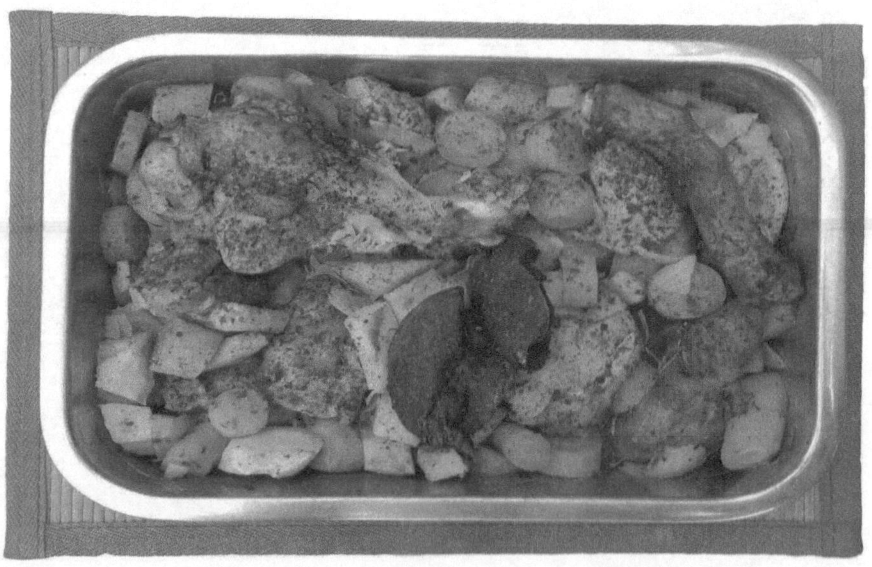

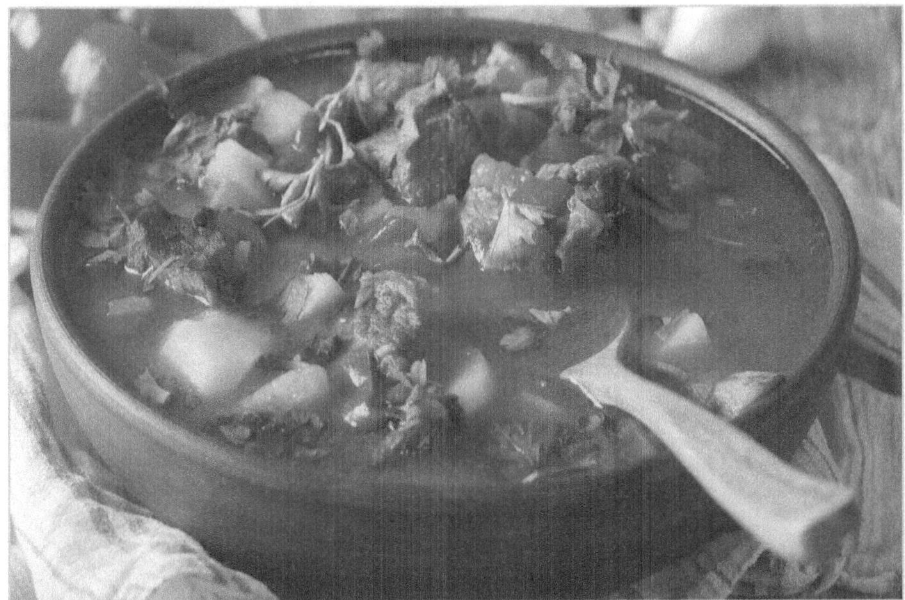

15- Goulash Soup Hungarian-Style (for one person)

- 400-600g of well-washed leg of beef
- 1 teaspoon sea salt
- 1 teaspoon freshly ground black pepper
- 150-250g chopped red onion
- 1-2 tablespoons slightly hot red pepper powder
- 2 garlic cloves, crushed
- 1 tomato, chopped
- 2 bay leaves
- 1 teaspoon of cumin
- 200-300g carrot, finely chopped
- 100-150g parsnip, finely chopped
- 100g celery, finely chopped

First, cut off the fat from the beef and melt the fat in a thick-bottomed ceramic frying pan, heating it up slowly. Dice the beef and add the salt and ground black pepper. Pour off the excess fat and from the ceramic frying pan, then add the chopped onion and the garlic, then simmer until the onion is transparent. Then remove the pan from the stove and stir in the red pepper powder.

Pour the resulting mixture and the beef into a thick-bottomed pot, and stirring constantly, heat it until the beef turns a lighter whitish color. Then pour boiling water into the pan to cover the beef and add the tomatoes and bay leaves.

Put the cumin into a filter and immerse it in the beef stew and simmer the goulash for 90-120 minutes. Then remove the filter of cumin and add the carrot, parsnip and celery. Bring to the boil, then lower the heat, cover and stew for 50 additional minutes.

16- Agard-Style Fisherman's soup

- 400-600g of fish
- 1 tablespoon chopped parsley
- 1 tablespoon chopped celery leaf
- 500g of carrots, parsnips and celery

Start cooking fish with parsley and celery leaf for a traditional fisherman's soup with little water and without any thickening for a few minutes, and then add the vegetables for a further 40 minutes of cooking, such as carrot, parsnip and celery to taste.

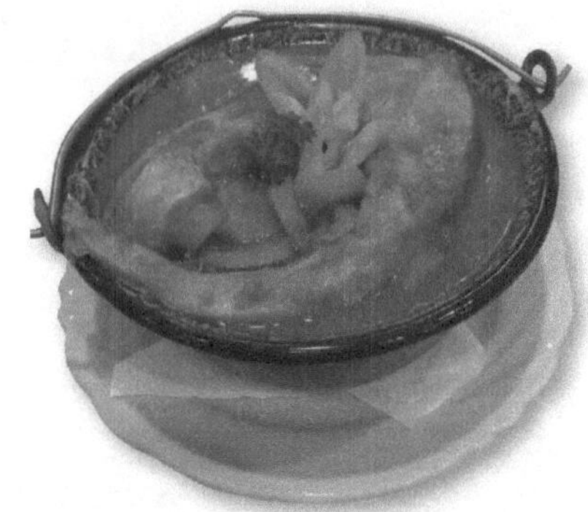

17- Chili Beans and Other Vegetable Pottages

If possible, cook chili beans and other vegetable pottages from freshly podded leguminous plants. If there are none available, soak desiccated leguminous plants for a couple of hours. While braising the pottage, you should thicken it with dry roux (Recipes 18) or a thickening agent (Recipes 19). Otherwise, prepare vegetable pottages in the traditional way.

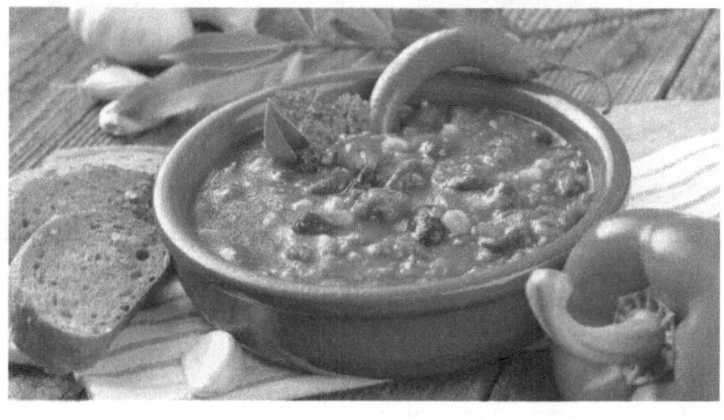

18- Dry Roux Thickening Mix

- 1-2 tablespoons wholegrain flour
- 1-2 cloves of garlic
- paprika powder to taste

Spread a little vegetable oil across the surface of a thick-bottomed ceramic frying pan, heat it for a minute and then wipe the excess oil off the surface with a paper towel. Then add the finely-chopped garlic and simmer on a low heat for a little while, stirring with a plastic or wooden kitchen spoon constantly. When it is ready, sprinkle the wholegrain flour evenly over the garlic in the pan and brown it slightly, stirring and shaking it constantly. Then taking the pan off the stove, sprinkle the paprika onto the mix and stir in, and then add some water making it a smooth paste.

If you are cooking chili beans, add the chili with the paprika.

19-Thickening Agent

Cooking with a thickening agent should be done in the traditional way. But, instead of using sour cream or milk, stir the wholegrain flour into soy milk or soy yogurt.

Blood group O and B individuals should use wholegrain oat flour instead of wheat flour. Dishes prepared with dry roux contains no oil, therefore no unnecessary calories and trans-fats.

20- Vegan broth

Any leguminous plant and any vegetable that may be cooked are suitable for this meal. Based on your preference, many types of flavoring, and dry roux (Recipes 18) or thickening liaison (Recipes 19) are applicable. It is important to prepare the soup to as thick as possible since the thinner the soup is the harder it is to digest it as it dilutes the digestive juices.

21- Coconut Ball Cookie (for 4 people)

- 250g of brown rice
- 1 liter / 2 pints of water or soy or almond milk
- 2-4 tablespoons tapioca or corn starch or 1-2 packets of chocolate pudding powder
- 200-300g thin-rolled whole oats
- 10-15 tablespoons cocoa powder
- 60-80 stevia tablets
- desiccated coconut crumbs

Cook the rice in plenty of water (Recipes 2) When it is cooked, add the water or soy or almond milk, as well as the tapioca or corn starch or chocolate pudding powder. Work it to a smooth mixture with a strong hand blender. Bring it to the boil again, and add the rolled whole oats and stir until it reaches a thick paste. Then mix together well with the cocoa powder and 60-80 stevia tablets, dissolved in a little water. Allow the mixture to cool somewhat.

Then form 4-5 cm balls from the hot thick paste, and roll them in coconut crumbs.

This is an excellent dessert, and if you have a sweet tooth, it may be even your main dish. This cookie may be consumed by diabetic people; it contains no sugar but only slowly absorbed complex carbohydrates and precious nutriments. Thus you may dine on as many coconut balls as you wish; you will not gain excess weight, only your muscles will be stronger.

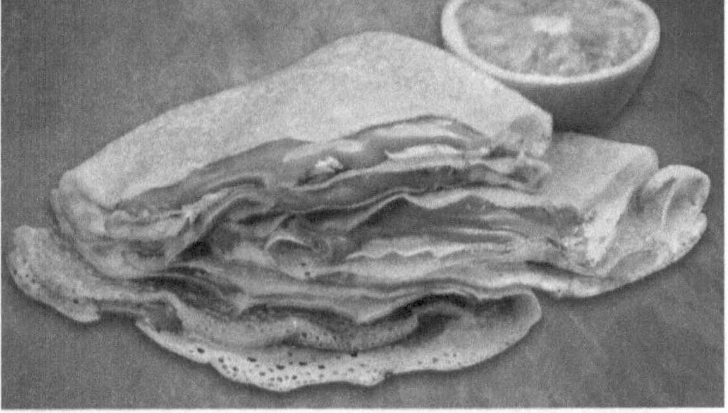

22-Pancake

The following ingredients are required for 5 pancakes:

- 6 tablespoons wholegrain oat flour
- 3 tablespoons buckwheat flour
- 2 tablespoons tapioca or corn starch
- pinch of sea salt
- pinch of baking soda
- a little sugar or natural sweetener

Mix the ingredients together well with 0.5 liter / 1 pint cold water or soy or almond milk to taste using an electric blender, then leave the resulting smooth pancake batter in the fridge for half a day. If necessary, you can thicken it with a little oatmeal or thin it by adding a little soda.

Fry the pancake in a thick-bottomed ceramic frying pan with the least possible coconut oil or butter.

23- Ceramic Pan-Frying Tofu

Slice some good-quality tofu to half an inch thick, or cut it into half-inch cubes. Spread a teaspoon of cold-pressed vegetable oil or butter on the surface of a thick-bottomed ceramic frying pan, heat it up and wipe the excess oil or butter off the surface with a paper towel. Fry the tofu slices or cubes on a low heat for 20 minutes, turning the cubes continuously. The slices should be turned over once after 10 minutes' frying.

24- Sweet-Sour or Szechuan tofu

Pour sweet and sour or Szechuan sauce into the thick-bottomed ceramic frying pan over the freshly fried hot tofu (Recipes 23) Bring to the boil and cook together for a minute. Once cooled, add some honey and possibly some freshly chopped chili and onion. You can prepare this sauce, but for speed, use good-quality canned sauce that is made without artificial preservative.

25- Vegan Pizza

If you do not want to bother with making the pizza dough you can buy ready-to-cook pizza dough that is made from wholegrain flour suitable for your blood group, and does not contain egg. Spread tomato sauce on over the pizza base, and sprinkle it with oregano, basil, leguminous plants, vegetables and some soy cheese to taste. If you are not worried about gaining weight, you can use mozzarella. This creamy cheese is very unhealthy and fattening and has very low protein content, thus in small quantities, it is digestible as fat.

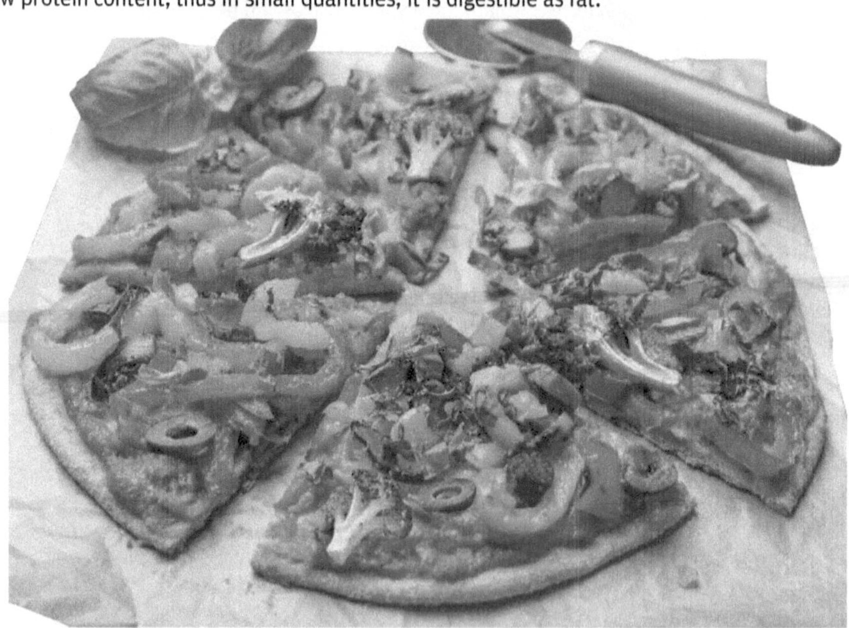

26- Vegan Hamburger

Similar to vegan pizza, buy or bake hamburger rolls that are made from wholegrain flour which suits your blood group, and does not contain egg. As you prefer, place lettuce, sliced red onion, sliced tomato or any other vegetable between the hamburger breads.

You can add chili sauce or ketchup although you should know that ketchup is unhealthy due to its boiled tomatoes, vinegar and sugar, even if artificial preservatives are not used for preparation. If you decide to consume it, try the chili version, as chili makes its taste stronger thus a smaller quantity is enough for sufficient flavoring. Use vegan tartare sauce instead of mayonnaise.

Instead of meat, put a large slice of well-seasoned breaded eggplant into the hamburger (Recipes 4). You can likewise cook vegan patties from leguminous plants or bulbous vegetables which can be thickened with tapioca, oatmeal, or corn starch instead of egg. This should be flavored to taste with ground cumin, chili, black pepper, paprika, garlic, onion, basil, and oregano. If you desire beef hamburger, put some beef flavoring in the patty or the breading used for the eggplant. Artificial flavorings are unhealthy, but the harm is negligible if we flavor a healthy meal with them, instead of consuming a very unhealthy food.

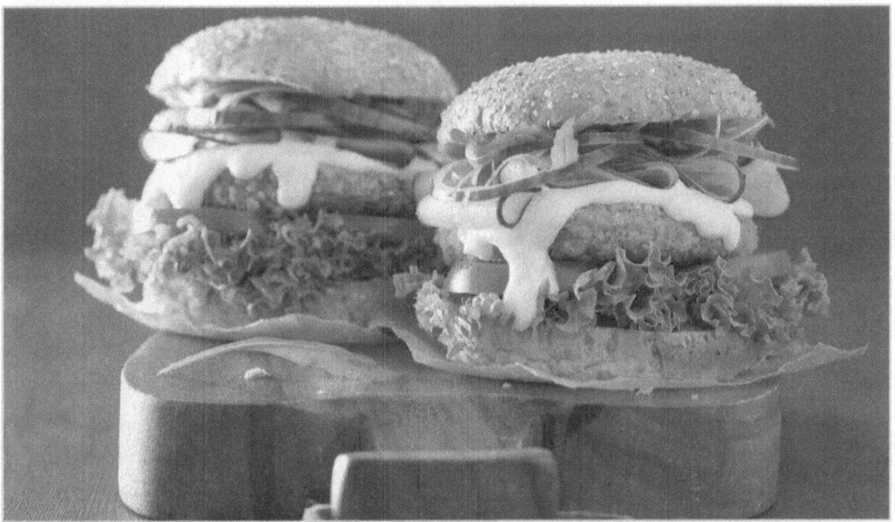

27- Brown Rice Pudding

Cook brown rice in a thick-bottomed pot (Recipes 2) with a little more water than usual. This way you do not need to worry too much about burning the rice, however pay attention to prevent foam boiling over from the pot, as the starch in it helps the pudding to firm. Then for each 500g of brown rice, add one tablespoon of ground cinnamon, 15-20 stevia tablets, and use a hand blender to mix them with half the amount of the hot rice. The resulting paste should be mixed with the other half of the rice, then pour all the rice into a flat rectangle-shaped cooking pan. Once it is cooled down, cut into squares and serve it with some jam to taste.

28- Chocolate Pudding (from brown rice milk)

 Cook brown rice in a large thick-bottomed cooking pot (Recipes 2) with more water than usual and for somewhat longer than usual. This way you do not need to worry too much about burning the rice. Pay attention to prevent the foam boiling over from the pan as the starch in it helps the pudding to firm. Once ready, for each 500g of brown rice add 0.3-0.4 liter / 10 fl oz of water or soy milk to taste and work it in thoroughly with a strong hand blender then add 40g good-quality rolled oats, 40-60 stevia tablets, 6-8 tablespoons cooking cocoa powder, and 1-2 tablespoons corn or tapioca starch. Instead of starch, you can add one packet of chocolate pudding powder. (Artificial flavorings in it are unhealthy, but the harm is negligible if we flavor a healthy meal with them, instead of faking the taste of a very unhealthy food.) Then work it again thoroughly with the hand blender to a smooth paste, bring to the boil again and then pour it into 4 bowls to chill.
The resulting pudding will be digested easily and satisfy your appetite since it contains only essential nutriments, for this it is incomparable with the traditional chocolate pudding.

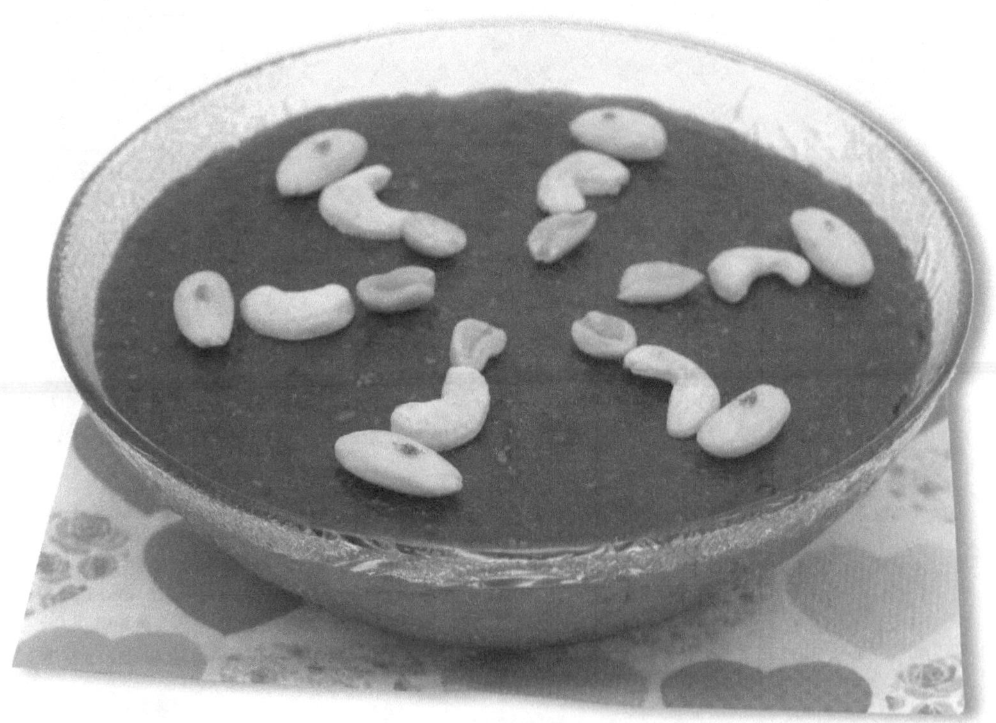

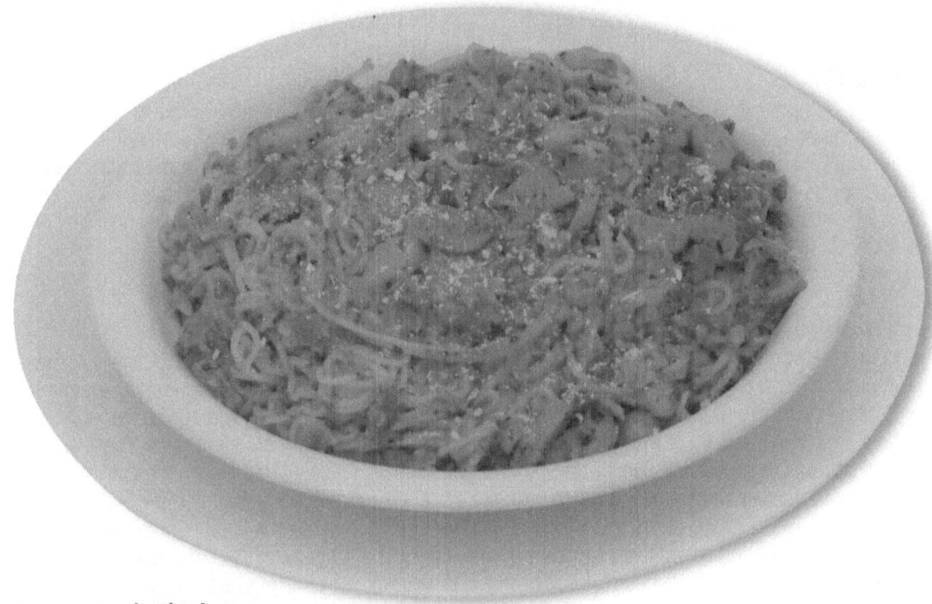

29- Vegan Spaghetti Bolognese

The following quantities are measured for two people.
- 100g carrot, finely chopped
- 100g parsnip, finely chopped
- 100g celery, finely chopped
- 200g red onion
- 2 garlic cloves, finely chopped
- pinch of sea salt
- 1 teaspoon ground cumin
- 1 teaspoon oregano
- 1 teaspoon basil
- 250-300g of canned or precooked chickpeas
- 400g canned or precooked Bolognese sauce

First, prepare the sauce. Use a thick-bottomed high-quality ceramic frying pan, large enough to fry everything at once. Place it on the largest hob in order to receive sufficient heat on all sides of the pan to make its surface evenly hot. Heat a teaspoon of extra virgin olive oil in the pan and make sure it spreads over the entire surface of the pan. Then you can wipe the oil off the pan with a paper towel.

Add the chopped carrot, parsnip and celery to the pan and sprinkle with black pepper. Brown gently for 15 minutes then add the onion and fry until it becomes transparent. Add the garlic, sea salt, cumin, oregano and basil and fry for a further 2 minutes. Then add the canned or pre-cooked chickpeas and crush them with a plastic or wooden kitchen spoon. Then add the Bolognese sauce. Bring it to the boil and simmer for 5 minutes.

Cook 200g durum or rice pasta according to your blood type, following the instructions written on the packaging of the pasta. Once ready, serve the pasta into dishes and pour the sauce over it, then serve with a sprinkle of Parmesan cheese. This hard cheese is very unhealthy and fattening and has a very low protein content, thus in small quantities it is digestible as fat.

Conclusion

Our Environment

Unfortunately, due to years of environmental pollution, the ozone layer surrounding the Earth has become thinner and hollow, therefore it does not filter the ultraviolet radiation which damages our unprotected eyes very quickly. So when outdoors, you should wear sunglasses or UV-B filtering eyeglasses, if you do not want to have to wear always prescription glasses for your damaged eyes later in life. Unfortunately, neither clouds nor water vapor filter UV radiation, therefore it is just as damaging in cloudy weather.

Misled by Industries

Nowadays the pharmaceutical and food industries are the most profitable in the world. They are owned by some of the wealthiest men on Earth who are capable of doing anything for money. Their interest is to produce food from the cheapest ingredients, even if the result is unhealthy to our bodies or harmful to the planet, and filled with synthetic flavorings in order to improve their original taste. These artificial additives cause a type of addiction.

These people spend a lot of money on advertising to market the higher commercial traffic of their well-flavored products. For example, they hire healthy-looking child actors to consume milk chocolate or other junk food while running and playing happily with older people. By watching this commercial, in our subconscious, each of us connects health, happiness and long life to the consumption of this kind of product, due to the way our brain processes what we see. Also, when we taste them, they seem to be incredibly delicious due to artificial flavorings in them. Based on these sensations, our subconscious makes the assumption that these substances are excellent and healthy for us.

Our tongue distinguishes four basic tastes which our subconscious uses to identify the type of food we consume. These are the salty flavor such as found in meat; intensely sweet flavor such as in fruit; moderately sweet such as complex carbohydrates (seeds, grains used to make bread products and so on); sour such as spoiled food which has begun to ferment; bitter such as poisonous food and we should avoid. But this identification process works only if the original taste is not modified by synthetic flavors. Nobody would voluntarily drink rapeseed oil or palm oil since the horrible flavor would immediately tell their subconscious that these oils are inconsumable. However, if the taste of these foodstuffs is improved by synthetic flavorings and sugar and their state is transformed to trans-fat by hydrogenation, these can be sold as chocolate for a higher price.

Our highly developed brains are able to analyze and form conclusions from our daily experiences in life, but our decisions are always determined by our subconscious, based on its stored images and our instincts. Thus, if our brain was not manipulated by commercials, then thanks to instructions from the subconscious, parents would consider the following points when considering buying chocolate for their kids: first, what is chocolate and what is it made from? Second, is it harmful or beneficial for the kids? Third, even if it is beneficial, should they buy for this price? I think the decision would be obvious. However, due to intense commercials and synthetic flavors, when we are purchasing these products, our subconscious does not instruct the conscious mind to perform a rational analysis of the situation. Hence, the brain makes an immediate decision based on artificially created images and flavors, perceiving chocolate as an excellent product that will make children run and play healthily and happily, living for long as the older actors in the commercials. This decision is the exact opposite of the result of conscious analysis. Ordinary people usually seek the best for their children instinctively, not even guns would make them feed poison to their children. Only commercials and synthetic flavors are able to do this job by tricking the subconsciousness. If children are fed with junk food, they will become addicted to it due to synthetic chemical ingredients, and will be on course for slowly developing type 2 diabetes and cardiovascular diseases or cancer.

Once someone consumes a sufficiently high amount of these artificial products and becomes sick, they will have to take medications and other treatments, thereby further enriching the aforementioned wealthiest people. Medical universities were built and are maintained by the donations of the pharmaceutical industry, and they also give out scholarships.

Studies

Moreover, the study materials of these universities are actually determined by their owners. For example, in experiments such as those conducted on rabbits in 1913 by Nikolay Anichkov, (which, unlike humans, are completely herbivorous.) Anichkov fed rabbits on egg yolk and pure cholesterol. In subsequent autopsies it was found that the veins and arteries of rabbits were calcified.

Based on this experiment, the pharmaceutical industry claimed that cholesterol causes calcification and cardiovascular diseases for humans. Following this falsehood, the food industry proclaimed margarine to be heart-friendly, even though butter does not contain any cholesterol. Nowadays it is commonly known that margarine is made from cheap hydrogenated vegetable oil that has been transformed into trans-fats, which does contribute towards cardiovascular diseases. For this reason, margarine is now taxed highly and cannot be promoted as a "healthy" alternative to butter in many countries.

The Myth of Cholesterol

It is a common fact that fat-soluble vitamins K1 and D3 are essential for absorbing calcium and are found in high-cholesterol foods such as egg yolk, liver and other animal offal. Arteriosclerosis, the hardening of the arteries, is caused by unabsorbed calcium stuck on the walls of veins and arteries. Up-to-date research and statistics prove that people with high cholesterol level have 0% chance of developing cardiovascular diseases, contrary to what we have been told for many years. Furthermore, since cholesterol-lowering pills have been prescribed by doctors (worth billions of dollars) to prevent cardiovascular diseases, the number of these diseases has actually multiplied. Therefore, the health and life of the whole population of the Earth are seriously threatened.

As a lay-person, I wonder how it is possible that nobody in the pharmaceutical industry has ever thought to experiment on animals that usually substitute humans in similar experiments, such as pigs or rats rather than herbivorous rabbits. By feeding them egg yolk, liver and other animal offal, we could observe whether these cause arteriosclerosis and cardiovascular diseases in them.

Furthermore, it would be worth reading statistics about the people who take cholesterol-lowering medication and see if they subsequently develop cardiovascular diseases. Unfortunately, however, these statistics are as yet confidential, and for this reason, I can only bring up a personal example of my father and myself.

Some Personal Stories

My father was in perfect health in his youth, but his physician prescribed cholesterol- lowering medication for him to avoid cardiovascular diseases. A couple of years later he was diagnosed with heart disease, thus, besides the cholesterol-lowering medicine, he was given heart medicines and other pills. He has been treated with heart surgery four times, taking further pills for his recovery. Despite these treatments, he is continuously sick. In his case it is obvious that cholesterol-lowering medicines did not protect him from heart disease. My father is stubborn and already in his later years and believes that eating habits have no correlation with his health, thus it is hard to convince him to change his lifestyle.

According to the current statistics, high cholesterol is a 100% protecting factor against cardiovascular diseases. Therefore, using our common sense, if this is lowered by "medicines", then this protection is removed, giving way to cardiovascular diseases and to their medications.

These statistics are valid for the European and American populations, where the majority of people are blood group O. In the cases of blood group A and AB individuals, if their cholesterol is lowered by taking pills instead of avoiding liver-intake, toxins accumulated in the animal liver they consume may cause cancer.

Medical experts and physicians are rewarded by the pharmaceutical industry with exceptionally expensive holidays and trips, if they manage to prescribe a certain amount of medicine in a given period of time.

Consequently, if a person is suffering from viral influenza, which is a genetically modified fake virus, it is not surprising if, without a thorough inspection of the patient, the GP prescribes antibiotics which have no effect whatsoever on viral infections.

Only our own immune system is able to protect us from viruses, nothing else. However, its functioning can be strengthened by vaccines, healthy diets and by the daily consumption of 1-2 garlic cloves. Antibiotics do not do anything to any virus, only kill harmless bacteria and harm our natural immune system, and have led to the evolution of new strains of super-bacteria, which are completely resistant to every antibiotic.

I would not like to write further about tougher topics, but you should not expect real health from your physician, only pills, vaccines, and treatments will be prescribed. The symptoms of sicknesses and diseases that have developed due to unsatisfactory eating habits are well treated with these substances, however, by hiding the real issue of bad eating habits, they usually cause other health problems and diseases. Of course, new pills and treatments follow and the cycle continues. If you live in the UK, you do not need to worry so much as the NHS is a good system. However, you can only be really healthy by maintaining an appropriate diet, nothing else.

Do not get me wrong, if you are sick, go to your GP, but it is better to avoid such situations. I used to be sickly during my childhood and had to take a lot of medication, but my condition became worse and worse. Hence, stronger pills were prescribed, but my condition diminished further; I gained excess weight and spent months in hospitals where I was diagnosed with a number of diseases. Of course, they prescribed different medicines for all of them.

By the age of seven, due to processed foods and medications, my obesity reached such a level that I could not even step up on a stool during physiotherapy. By this time, besides my high cholesterol level, I was treated for heart disease, infectious mononucleosis, rheumatic fever, and several viral and bacterial infections. Recovering from flu was impossible or took several months, and then I was healthy only for a couple of days. Of course, one sneeze meant a visit to the GP and new pills that I had to take with my mother's assistance.

The doctors claimed that my natural immune system was not functioning so I had to take 10 antibiotics pills a day. Depending on the seriousness of my diseases, my intake of pills varied between 20-30 a day. My condition diminished further and before long, I ended up in the emergency room. My electrocardiography (ECG) results showed that my heart was in horrible condition and my life was in immediate danger. By chance, one of the nurses noticed that I never finished the meat and vegetables served for lunch and dinner and told me to eat them as they would make me stronger. I told her I didn't like the meat as it smelled bad, thus I received a double portion of chicken instead of pork, which I ate with vegetables. I recovered in one week.

I was released from hospital and went home, where nobody told me to eat meat and vegetables or observed the quantity of my chocolate and cookie consumption. Consequently, I ended up in hospital again, where the advice of the nurse came back to my mind, making me more conscious of my eating habits. I recovered again in only a couple of days.

Since it become obvious to me by the age of 9 that pills always sent me to hospital, while just healthy nutrition could set me free, I started visiting bookshops and bought all the books I could find about eating and nutritional science. I started studying them while following a healthy eating habit. My condition improved drastically, even though I made plenty of mistakes by then.

A year later, I decided not to take any chemicals (known as medication) any more. Of course, my physician was worried and thought I might die. He tried to convince me to take at least the cholesterol-lowering medication, as my cholesterol level reached an extremely high level as soon as I stopped taking them, possibly causing heart attack in a couple of weeks. I had to sign a few documents to show that I had quit the treatments of my own free will. One month later I was still alive, moreover, with improved strength and physical condition.

My test results improved a lot except my high cholesterol level, which was so high that my death was due in a couple of days (according to the doctors). Analyzing my chances, we concluded that if were fortunate enough not to die from a heart attack, I might live up to forty years. I had no way of knowing whether this was true, however by then my wellbeing had improved to such a level that I began to think that living only for twenty years might be better than further suffering endless medications and treatments for the next thirty years. At that age, I still did not understand what he was talking about, but I knew that the huge quantities of pills I had been taking only sent me to the emergency room, from where I could only recover by healthy eating. Thus, I told my doctor to leave me alone and stopped going to my check-ups.

I went back one year later, when they confirmed that I had no heart disease, and my rheumatic fever and mononucleosis infection were likewise gone. They concluded that I had been misdiagnosed for these diseases as it is impossible for them to go away without treatments. (By the way, are you aware of the main cause of death in the US, where the healthcare system is the best in the world for compensations? It is not cancer, heart attack, or accidents, but misdiagnosis.)

I have not taken any pills ever since, not just out of principle. I have been sick only once when I was infected by H1N2 bird flu virus, from which I recovered without medication, only experiencing slight sneezing and fever for 2-3 days. Also, I have been doing sports for 36 years, and now, at the age of 46, I am in perfect health, even though I have rather lived a somewhat debauched life.

A couple of years ago I visited my physician for a medical examination, knowing without a doubt that I had no health-related problems. When I received my blood-test results, my physician told me that my cholesterol level was high and my 110/70 blood pressure was low. To treat them, she prescribed cholesterol-lowering and blood pressure-increasing medication. The day before, I had run a half-marathon, and my usual 120/80 blood pressure was lower the following day as I was resting.

The physician did not check my blood pressure again to see whether it stabilized to its normal state before prescribing the medication. Fortunately, I already knew from statistics that as long as my cholesterol level is high, I am 100% protected from all cardiovascular diseases, from which I had already recovered once when I was eight years old and had stopped taking cholesterol-lowering medication. Reacting to this, the physician explained that my life was in great danger, thus I wavered. Had I not been studying this specific field for 36 years, I would have taken the recommended medicines as the lady seemed to be a caring person and a firm believer in the medications and treatments she had studied at university.

Take Responsibility for Your Own Health

In the US, due to lawsuits and compensations, physicians no longer prescribe cholesterol-lowering medications. Thus, the pharmaceutical industry there, since the occupation of Afghanistan, opened a new front to distribute heroin-like opium derivatives, creating sleeping pills, painkillers, and tranquilizers. People taking these substances develop an opium addiction for a lifetime, without being aware of its dangers when they first start to take them.

Consumers take a large number of these extremely expensive pills (even heroin) in many cases, after intense suffering. But this does not help for long. Of course, this process affects the health negatively, which means a new market for further medicines, vaccines, and needles. These facts remind me of the Trojan Horse rather than of Hippocrates, who was famous for his quote "Let food be your medicine and medicine be your food," long before the Hippocratic oath came into being. Many have been tricked into believing that everything can be cured with pills. You should not forget that modern medicine is not a science with as long a history as mathematics and physics, which have been developing for more than 2000 years.

Until 1942, when the first antibiotic Penicillin became available, medicine mainly constituted using old-fashioned but expensive treatments such as leeches to draw blood. Although methodologies have advanced significantly, the point remained the same: to merchandize products. It is of less importance whether the products are a modern substance or leeches; the point is to increase sales and maximize profits. Accordingly, I would caution everybody not to trust this newly-founded science as much as disciplines with long traditions, whose practitioners have been observing reality and experimenting, discovering correlations and observing patterns or trends without increasing their wealth and lying about their researches. Medical science is a recent discipline, which, without human experiments that are prohibited, gropes in the dark. Some fields such as surgery are exceptions, but the pharma industry is a

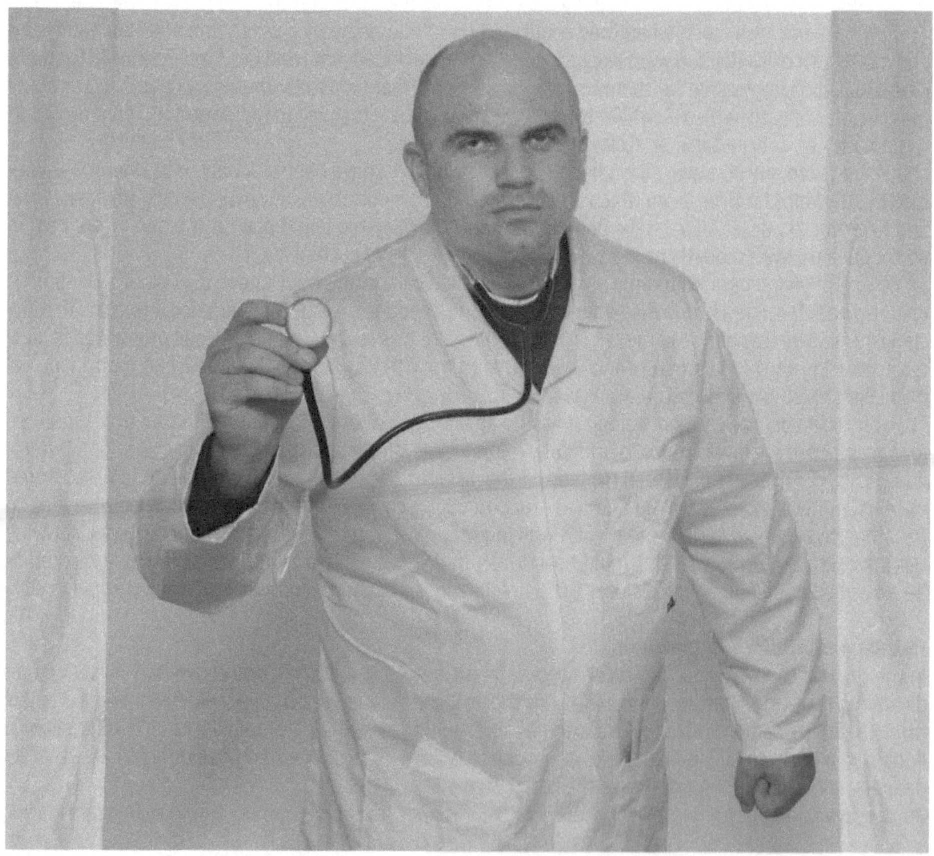

dead end. It is not only unable to cure most illnesses completely, but in many cases, the pharmaceutical industry has no solution whatsoever.

As long as we eat healthily, we will be in good physical shape and need not worry about obesity. Although doctors have taken the Hippocratic oath, they are taught little about nutrition other than the amount of bread diabetics can consume per day and what kind of medication is required for this level of wheat consumption. For this reason, it is not even mentioned by doctors that people with diabetes must avoid any consumption of white roll or bread since type 2 diabetes is caused by the sugar content of wheat, and other carbohydrates should be advised.

And besides nutrition, Hippocrates taught that sport and good humor are essential for health. For medication, he and his students mainly used marihuana and in some cases, they used cocaine. The active agent of marihuana is the Delta-9 tetrahydrocannabinol which is a very effective medicine against about half of the existing human diseases, for example against AIDS, glaucoma, multiple sclerosis, pain suffered by paraplegics and quadriplegics and many others, and is the only existing, really effective medicine against all kinds of cancers and all psychiatric diseases including epilepsy and Parkinson's Disease.

Delta-9 tetrahydrocannabinol is the only painkiller and sedative which, when taken orally, has no side effects at all. However, after pressure from the drug industries Delta-9 tetrahydrocannabinol was prohibited in Europe and in the American continent where ordinary people did not know anything about marihuana.

Ironically, since then, experts in the pharmaceutical industry have been trying to innovate an artificial version of Delta-9 tetrahydrocannabinol, yet they have failed, despite the fact that the human brain possesses all the necessary receptors for the Delta-9 tetrahydrocannabinol, proving the long-term consumption of it by humans is safe. Regrettably, the doctor-patient relationship is similar to any business connection, where the two sides have opposing interests. Patients would like to be healthy while spending the least amount of money possible for recovery, while the pharmaceutical industry relies on sick people with long-term medication needs in order to be the richest industry on Earth. The more people seek drugs and medication, the more money will be amassed by the few richest people selling those drugs. This amounts to about 18% of the entire world trade. Moreover, it is the most profitable business on Earth without taking in to account the additional expenditure on trade chains, advertising and transportation for the size and weight of the products. Your interests are best served by observing the principles explained in this book.

Since the publication of blood group diet books, I have not been able to obtain any information about my blood type from my general practitioner and from other doctors. Maybe you will be lucky, and you can find it written on your birth certificate.

Good books on this subject have been published before with some inaccuracies, however, these presented this complex topic only from the perspective that the author found important. Therefore, these often demanded unhealthy and unnecessary self-torture from the reader. And, they make it difficult to understand why a diet is promoted as healthy or otherwise as these books only served 20-30% of the required information about this very complex issue.

The best books on this topic in my opinion, have been "Fit for Life" from Harvey and Marilyn Diamond, "Eat Right 4 your Type" by the D'Adamo family, and books about the macrobiotic diet. The Paleo diet was not a bad idea for blood group O individuals at its beginning, but it went off-track. A really effective alternative has not been proposed until now.

This book provides a brief and simple explanation about everything important from all perspectives; thus, you don't need to read unnecessary or false information about anything. This book is 100% checked and verified, and without unnecessary prohibitions, suggests the optimal diet for you according to your blood type. As long as you observe it, you will be in perfect health.

See our website: www.perfectselfcontrol.com

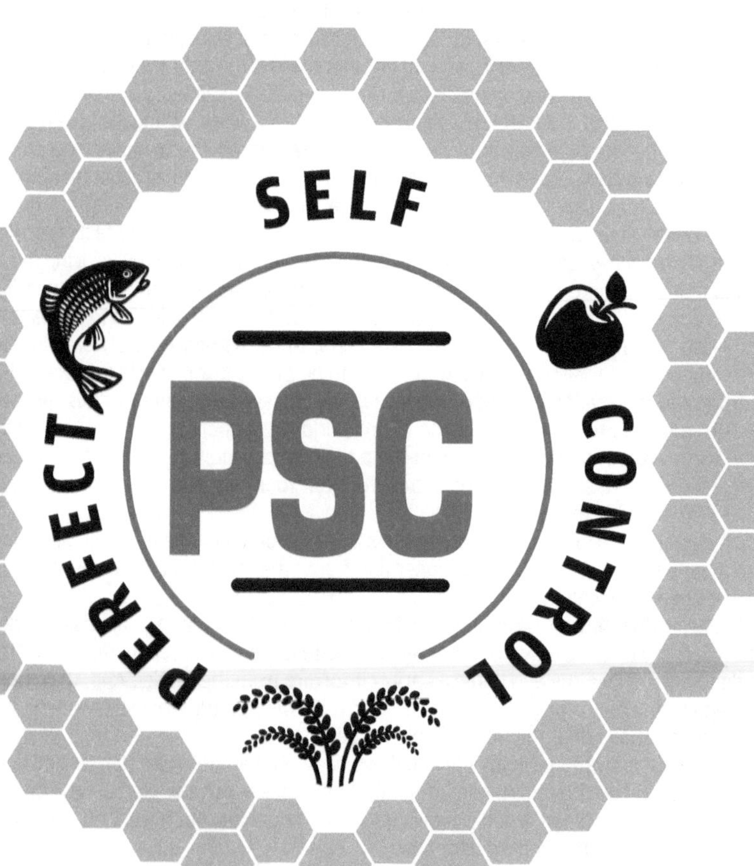

SELF
PSC
PERFECT
CONTROL